Marisa Peer studied hypnotherapy at the Hypnotism Training Institute of Los Angeles, known as the best hypnotherapy training establishment in the world. She has spent over twenty-five years working with an extensive client list, including royalty, rock stars, actors, CEOs and professional and Olympic athletes. Marisa has developed her own unique style, which is frequently referred to as life-changing. Her previous books, *You Can Be Thin* and *Ultimate Confiden*　　　　 published in 2007 and 2009.

Marisa also studied with Deepak Chopra and at the Pritikin Longevity Center in California and trained in Cell Command Therapy, a proven technique that commands cells to age more slowly. She works extensively on television and radio, and has appeared on *Supersize vs. Superskinny* and *Celebrity Fit Club* UK and USA. Marisa featured in Tatler's *Guide to Britain's 250 Best Doctors* and was voted Best British Therapist. She gives lectures and workshops all over the world.

Visit her website at *www.marisapeer.com*.

WITHDRAWN

YOU
CAN BE
YOUNGER

MARISA PEER

HIGH LIFE HIGHLAND	
3800 14 0030281 0	
Askews & Holts	Apr-2014
613.019	£13.99

piatkus

WITHDRAWN

PIATKUS

First published in Great Britain in 1997 by Michael Joseph Ltd as *Forever Young*
This updated and revised version first published 2014 by Piatkus

Copyright © 2014 Marisa Peer

The moral right of the author has been asserted.

All rights reserved.
No part of this publication may be reproduced, stored in a
retrieval system, or transmitted in any form or by any means, without
the prior permission in writing of the publisher, nor be otherwise circulated
in any form of binding or cover other than that in which it is published
and without a similar condition including this condition
being imposed on the subsequent purchaser.

A CIP catalogue record for this book
is available from the British Library.

ISBN 978-0-349-40282-6

Typeset in Sabon by M Rules
Printed and bound in Great Britain by
Clays Ltd, St Ives plc

Papers used by Piatkus are from well-managed forests
and other responsible sources.

MIX
Paper from
responsible sources
FSC   FSC® C104740
www.fsc.org

Piatkus
An imprint of
Little, Brown Book Group
100 Victoria Embankment
London EC4Y 0DY

An Hachette UK Company
www.hachette.co.uk

www.piatkus.co.uk

To download the free hypnosis sessions that accompany this book,
visit www.marisapeer.com/ycby-audio-download.

This book is dedicated to the memory of the
very special Audrey Pasternak, who truly defied ageing.
Darling Audrey we all miss you but because you live
on in our hearts you won't ever be forgotten.

It is also dedicated to my wonderful husband
John – you are the funniest, nicest, kindest, most
appreciated husband; you make me feel loved every day –
and to my gorgeous daughter Phaedra, who keeps
me young and happy in every possible way.

Contents

Acknowledgements

First, huge thanks to my husband John, who is so supportive of everything I do and does everything to make my life easier – thank you for making me so happy.

Thank you to all my family: to my beautiful daughter Phaedra and to Bree, Lucas, Carlyss, Freya and Isaac, for so much unconditional love and for always filling me up with love and laughter; to Sian, for being such a special and wonderful sister; to my dad Ron Peer, who taught me all the right things; to my mum Dee and to Cissie, because you gave me everything.

Very special thanks and acknowledgements to all my amazing friends: to Claudia Rosencrantz, Daniela Neumann, Helen Barbour and Mark Stoker, Jessica Richards, Charles Montagu, Philippa Hardman, Les and Glyn Robinson and Maria and Gordon Thomson – thank you for reading and re-reading my manuscripts, for supporting me, motivating me, endorsing me and, most of all, for believing in me and this book. I feel so blessed to have friends like you.

To my very own Peer group – thank you for the Peer Pressure, it's so good.

To my agent Claudia Webb and my editor Anne Lawrence for all your guidance.

To Rosie Spinks for being an indispensable PA.

To Dr Susan Horsewood Lee for her ongoing and much appreciated support.

And to my own teachers, especially the remarkable late Gil Boyne, none of this would exist if I had not been fortunate enough to meet you: you changed my life and I will never forget it.

'If one person breathes easier on the planet because of you, your life has a purpose.' And all of the above people do that for me all the time, so thank you.

And most especially to you, for having the desire to change, to slow down ageing – this book was written for *you*.

INTRODUCTION

'For each age is a dream that is dying, or one that is coming to birth'

Arthur William Edgar O'Shaughnessy 1844–81

There are many books already published promising to show you how to look younger, but this one is different. The current anti-ageing books available persuade you to change how you dress or how you eat or the products you use in order to look younger. I am going to show you how to change the way you think and what you do in order to not only look and feel younger but to also physically become younger. *You Can Be Younger* shows you how to look and feel ten years younger in a matter of weeks. Believe me, it really is possible to see results that quickly. In fact, you can look and feel younger in even less time than that.

Surprised? Well consider this: have you ever gone away for a week-long holiday, or even for a long weekend, only to return to hear people telling you that you look younger? Have you ever noticed that when one of your friends is newly in love she looks younger and better, or even radiant? Or perhaps you have noticed that when you have enjoyed wonderful sex with your partner you look radiant, and even when you laugh, have fun or dance to some music you love, you begin to look and feel better?

The reason for this is because humans are designed in a way that makes particular things that we do communicate directly with our mind and body, telling us that we are young or even becoming younger. When we communicate to our bodies in this way we can literally begin to reverse and slow down ageing, and become younger. It isn't just about what we do but also what we think, say and feel that communicates to our body this same age-reversal response. In this book I will take you through the different ways you can communicate verbally and non-verbally to your mind in order to become younger. I will show you that these effects are neither temporary nor do they wear off, because you are about to change your thinking in an easy and compelling way that will have a permanent and wonderful effect on your body. You will learn how to use this to your advantage further in this book.

Do you believe that ageing is something that is just going to happen to you? Do you feel that you can do nothing about it? Do you expect to lose your looks, your memory, your mental faculties and even your ability to move around easily? If you do, you really need this book. You have so much power to influence how you will age – a power you are not even aware of at the moment. You can hold on to your looks, your memory and your mobility, and you can grow older in years and yet look, feel and act younger. I promise you that just days into this programme you can feel so different and, instead of viewing getting older with fear and dread, you will be able to take charge of how you age so that you get older fabulously without growing old.

We live in a very ageist society. People are categorised according to their age, and we are becoming more preoccupied with how old we feel, how old we look and how old we are. One of the reasons for this preoccupation with ageing is because we are living longer and are physically younger than our predecessors were at the same age. Just a few hundred years ago the life expectancy was, in general, below 50 years of age, and life was much harder. People who lived beyond 50 were tired and their bodies were worn out. Living a long life and looking young was certainly not a priority for most people, but so much has changed in a relatively short time. Now, 50 is young, and at 50 you can be only halfway through your life. A person who is 50 years old today will have quite a different body from a 50-year-old from the 1900s. In fact, a 50-year-old body today would, comparatively speaking, have the body of a 35-year-old from that era – I will go into this in more detail later. Right now I want you to understand that we are more preoccupied with ageing because of all the wonderful possibilities open to us that allow us to grow older yet remain younger.

After reading *You Can Be Younger* you will know how to look and feel younger at any age and at every stage of your life; you will begin to see why some people age too quickly and others really are forever young.

People who age very well and who remain young, leave clues. We all know someone who looks fantastic for their age and we can all find an example of someone who is active, agile and young in their eighties. Many of these people don't know exactly what it is they are doing that is keeping them young, but I do. I have made a career out of studying ageing and the mind's ability to slow it down, and I am so excited about sharing my knowledge with you. As you learn what to do to become and stay young, you will be motivated to love doing it and to make it a lifelong habit. Soon you too will be one of those people others look at and refer to as a wonderful example of staying young.

The American comedian George Burns said, 'You can't stop yourself growing older but you sure can stop yourself growing old', and he was right. You can stop yourself from looking, feeling and acting old, and this book will show you how easy it is to do just that.

The techniques in *You Can Be Younger* are easy to adopt – you may actually find them the easiest and best changes you have ever made. It is a great investment for you, because it will change your life. By using this book you will be improving the quality of your life. You will be able to look and feel younger at every stage of your life; you can live longer and better, and feel great about yourself. Having good genes may add only three years to your lifespan, but the methods in this book will allow you to live longer and to stay mentally and physically active so that you can enjoy every year of your life.

One of my clients, a very successful actress, was told by her agent on her fortieth birthday that she was now too old for the part she was auditioning for and that she would have to lie about her age if she wanted to continue getting lead parts. I did some work with her and helped her change her belief so that she saw herself at 40 as very powerful, dynamic and strong. She went on to star in a very successful series where she played the lead love interest, and in fact, because she was 40, she got even more publicity. She was playing a strong, sexy, independent woman who knows who she is. Because the concept of sexy middle-aged women is still quite new in television, her programme generated a lot of interest.

Another client of mine wanted to have a baby and was told that at 44 she was too old and had left it too late to become a mother. In our sessions we looked at the fact that women having babies in their forties is not a new thing. In the past, when women were having very large families they continued having babies well into their forties. We also decided that biologically she was way below 40 and that she could use the power of her mind to ovulate young, healthy, grade-A eggs. Using her new belief system, she did indeed go on to have a healthy baby. She also had a very easy pregnancy and an easy birth.

Another of my clients at 50 felt very uncomfortable in his job, because his 35-year-old boss constantly made jokes about old people. He became worried that he was not sharp or quick enough to perform well at work and he was very scared of his memory declining. We changed these beliefs very quickly, and he came to see that his brain would go on working wonderfully – and so would his body – if he stimulated them in the right way. Just days into the programme he reported an improvement in his memory and in the way he felt about himself. He began to realise that his boss was simply expressing his own feelings of inadequacy around someone of my client's experience, and the comments ceased to bother him.

By reading this book – and listening to the scripts for becoming younger (see pages 154–5) – you will become just as inspired as my clients and you will have all the strategies you need to condition yourself, and absolutely allow yourself, to look and feel younger, both physically and mentally.

We all need to *know* that ageing is much more of a choice than we have been led to believe. Normal ageing has never been defined, so what we think of as normal ageing is nothing more than abnormal conditioning. Ageing is unique and individual for each of us and it not easily predicted. We have all met, or heard of, people who are old or burned out at 30, and others who are young at 80.

The science of ageing

All over the world, scientists are at work to discover what makes us age and how we can prevent it or slow it down. This is no longer the stuff of science fiction. It is real – you *can* slow down ageing, and I am going to show you how. There is so much new information available that will help you if you want to age more slowly.

I love life, and I want to live for as long as possible while enjoying a great quality of life, and I want to show you how to make this happen for you. A great deal is being discovered in the anti-ageing field, and there is so much to choose from. Scientists all over the world are making regular breakthroughs in the anti-ageing market. Today there are many things you could do to delay, reverse and defy ageing as we know it. You could invest in diet, vitamins, exercise, anti-ageing hormones such as melatonin and dihydroepiandrosterone (DHEA), or even use Mountain Air Therapy to slow down the ageing of your organs. Indeed, there is a wealth of treatments available to you, although some of them are expensive and time-consuming, and some have not been researched sufficiently to be proven safe.

There is, however, an anti-ageing product available to you that is free, absolutely safe and foolproof; it is easy to use and fun, and it gets fast and lasting results – and, importantly, it is so simple. You don't have to go out and buy this product, because you already own it – it is here within you, and it is your mind. Your mind and your ability to change your thinking about ageing can, and will, make you younger. I can promise you that by sticking with this programme you will get results. Everything you need to become younger is in this programme: the techniques you need to use to condition your mind to be younger are right here, laid out for you in an easy-to-follow format.

As well as learning techniques that will allow you to always look younger than your years, you can learn how to stay mentally sharp into your eighties, with a good memory. Do you already see getting older as a time when your body becomes fragile and you can no longer move around easily? None of these things have to happen to you. You can maintain muscle tone and continue to exercise into your eighties and beyond.

There are so many new possibilities that will change the way you age and the way you feel about ageing. If your desire is to look and feel younger for as long as possible and to grow older without *growing* old, then you are ready to take the next step, to take action to make it happen.

The most important tool for use in anti-ageing is the mind. The human mind is the most powerful healing force there is. No drug in the world can match it and if it were ever possible to build a computer equivalent to the human brain, it would take at least two buildings the size of the world's highest skyscrapers just to house it. The most important change you must make in order to look and feel younger is to change your thinking, because:

- Changing your thoughts can make you younger.
- Changing your thoughts can make you live longer.
- Changing your thoughts can make you physically look better.

- Changing your thoughts can make you retain a great memory into your nineties.
- Changing your thoughts can allow you to remain active, fit and healthy throughout your life.

I am passionate about anti-ageing and living a longer, better life, but all my work and research is backed up by data that shows us the mind's ability to create physical changes in *the body*. Tufts University Medical School ran a series of tests to prove that the power of thought can cause the body to become 5 to 12 years younger.[1]

Every step you take in the anti-ageing field must be accompanied by a belief that you *can slow down ageing and become younger*. Using vitamins, diet and exercise can only work, and indeed will work much better, if you also use the power of your mind and your belief system to become younger.

One of the reasons ageing is impossible to define is because our life expectancy is constantly increasing. In Roman times it was 28 years; at the beginning of the 20th century, life expectancy was 43 years for men, and 47 years for women, and only 10 per cent of the population lived to 65 years.

Today, life expectancy is moving towards 86 years for women, especially French and Japanese women, and 79 years for men. The record of living to 120 years was broken by a Frenchwoman, Jeanne Calment, who died in 1997 aged 122. In slightly over 50 years we have doubled our life expectancy, and it is rising rapidly. Every three months we add another month to our life expectancy – or every three years we add another year to our lifespan. Not only are people living longer but they also tend to have younger organs, so someone of 40 today cannot be compared with someone of 40 a hundred years ago, because their bodies and organs would be entirely different. They would also look very different. The 40-year-old of a hundred years ago would usually look old and tired, somewhat worn out, whereas the 40-year-old today can be so young that they might even pass for a 29-year-old.

In previous generations, staying young was not a priority, because people generally had harder lives. By the time they reached their fifties they may have wanted to retire and become sedentary, since life was about surviving, raising children, and having enough to eat and somewhere to live.

Things have changed so much in the modern era. Better housing and sanitation, better medicine, a greater variety of food, easier working conditions and a better means of transport all mean that we can now reach retirement age, although we don't necessarily feel like retiring – and why should we? We are not worn out, we still have a desire for life and we don't like being old, because of all the negative connotations that being old is supposed to have. We may not feel old or wish to be viewed as old.

Retirement no longer means the time when you wind down and prepare for your final years. Instead, it can mean another exciting chapter of life with so much we can be, do and enjoy. If we retire at 60 and live for another 30 years, we are only two-thirds of the way through our lives. Knowing this can give us the incentive we need to enjoy this stage and to see all the advantages it has to offer us. Since our lives are different now, we can and must age differently. Retiring from work is not retiring from life, and we can be older in years while remaining younger in attitude, with a younger body, a younger mindset and a zest and passion for life.

In 2011 the first of the baby-boom generation reached the age of 65. There are now more people between the ages of 55 and 65 than of any other age. By the year 2000 every third person in the job market was over 40, leading companies to rethink their ageist policies. Ageism exists in almost every area of sport, in the media, in the arts and in the workplace, but since we are all ageing differently and have vast potential to remain young as we become older in years, ageism will eventually become unacceptable. It is rife in the music business, but when the Rolling Stones performed in 2012 and Mick Jagger spent two and a half hours dancing and running across the stage at the age of 69 it did a lot to change our perception of what ageing is and what ageing looks like.

We are the first generation to hold on to youth as we age, and this is very exciting and something that we can continue to improve and benefit from, as long as we are given the specific information and instructions that will enable this to happen. This book will give you that information and instruction, and it will show you how to achieve this – how to become and remain younger throughout your life.

Prepare to be younger

If, like many people, you are concerned with ageing, then it's worth knowing the facts. Do you know that your body does not actually age in the way you think it does, because 98 per cent of the atoms in your body were not even there a year ago? The majority of cells in your body have the ability to renew them-selves, meaning you are constantly making a whole new body, and no matter what age you are, much of your body is just ten years old or less. If you live to the age of 95, the only three main areas of cells in your body that have lasted that length of time are in the brain, the heart muscles and the cells in your eyes. The majority of other cells in our bodies have the incredible ability to renew themselves. We even grow a new skeleton approximately every ten years.

Our bodies are in a state of constant change, and each tissue within the body is renewing itself according to its own timetable. Your stomach lining is renewed every five days due to constant use. The surface layer of your skin renews itself approximately every two weeks. The only reason we age at all is because our bodies contain so many specialised cells that over a very long period of time they can no longer undergo the rejuvenating influ-ence of cell division. We age because of eventual wear and tear within the un-dividing cells that repair the damage. When you learn, through this programme, to influence those cells, you can slow down ageing and its effects.

Our body is constantly rejuvenating:

- New skin is made every month.
- A new liver is made every six weeks.
- A new stomach lining is made every four to five days.
- Our taste-bud cells renew themselves every ten days.
- Our blood renews itself every month.
- Our eye cornea cells regenerate every 48 hours.
- The raw material of our DNA changes every six weeks.
- The cells within our bodies are always new.
- You make a completely new skeleton every ten years.

Even your heart renews itself. Researcher Piero Anversa found that heart muscle cells can renew themselves in a process that takes about 20 years.[2] In 1999 Jonas Frisen announced that his studies had found stem cells (which can create new cells) within the brain.[3] Our intestinal lining is covered with a substance called villi, which helps to absorb the nutrients into our bodies. Cells in the villi renew every three days.

Recent research suggests that some lung cells renew themselves. The cells on the lung's surface renew themselves every two to three weeks.

It takes between three and six years for us to have a completely new head of hair. The hair on our eyebrows and eyelashes is renewed a lot quicker, at six to eight weeks. The liver is known for its amazing capacity to repair and regrow itself. Liver cells have a lifespan of around 150 days. Seventy per cent of the liver can be removed during surgery and 90 per cent will grow back within two months.

Each one of us is unique and each person's body ages according to its own timetable, but we have a great deal of ability to influence this process.

When we are toddlers and young children we all tend to age the same way. A hundred six-year-old children would all have the same internal organs, the same heart, lungs, muscles and kidneys. A hundred 60-year-old adults, however, would have vastly different hearts, lungs, muscles, kidneys and other organs. Some would be younger than 60, some older, depending on their lifestyles and their ageing beliefs or expectations.

When an unidentified body is found and information is relayed to the public for identification purposes, a ten-year leeway in age span will always be given. The news item might, for example, describe a woman between the ages of 35 and 45, or a man between the ages of 50 and 60, because ageing is increasingly hard to define. How good are you at guessing someone's age exactly right? Just take a look at all the people around you. Can you guess their ages correctly?

Types of ageing

The age you are in years is irrelevant, because we have three ages and three different ways of measuring our age. We have:

1 A chronological age
2 A biological age
3 A psychological age

Our chronological age is the age on our birth certificate. We put all of our emphasis on this age, when in reality it is only a part of how old we are.

Our biological age is the age of our body and the age of our organs. Our internal organs and cells all age according to their own timetable, which can fluctuate greatly. People who meditate or are very calm, for example, have been proven to be 12 to 15 years younger biologically than they are chronologically. This means that their organs are younger in years than the age on their birth certificate. A runner may have a younger heart and lungs than his actual age. But organs can also be older than their owners, especially in people who live very stressful lives, who drink heavily, smoke or use drugs and over-use prescription drugs. A recent US study on a particular group of 35-year-olds showed that they all had livers of 50-year-olds due to their self-abusive lifestyles. People who take care of themselves almost always have younger organs. Women who have babies much later in life may have very young reproductive organs biologically rather than chronologically, while some very young women go through menopause too early, so their organs are biologically older although chronologically they are young.

You may remember the client I mentioned earlier who was able to conceive aged 44 after following this programme. Her doctor was amazed at how biologically young her body was. Another of my clients used my programme to visualise perfect eggs before her IVF treatment, and at the embryo transfer her embryologist took a photo of her embryo and said it was almost impossible for a woman of her age to have embryos of that quality.

Our psychological age is the age we feel, and this can change from moment to moment. Listening to music from the past, dancing, laughing, being childlike rather than childish, and splashing in puddles or giggling all cause us instantly to feel younger. This feeling sends a message to our bodies, which then literally begin to grow younger, making younger hormones and younger chemicals. This has been documented and proven many times.

Feeling stressed, on the other hand, causes us to feel and look older, and this feeling sends a very different message to our bodies, which then produce different chemicals. The result can be an acceleration of the ageing process.

When we are happy or relaxed we make different chemicals from the ones we make when we are unhappy or anxious, and these can age or rejuvenate us depending on our thinking. Your skin is a gland that responds to your thinking. When we fall in love we feel young, carefree and happy. Have you ever noticed how falling in love feels the same at any age, whether we are 17 or 70? The wonderful feeling of being in love sends positive messages to our organs. We feel and act younger, we seem to glow, our skin blooms and our immune system is boosted. We find ourselves singing out loud, dancing around the kitchen, smiling at strangers and generally feeling benevolent. It has been proven that people who have certain ailments such as skin conditions, migraines or joint pains, can become free of the symptoms when they are in the initial stages of falling in love.

In contrast, being depressed or grieving sends different messages to our organs with the result that we feel and act older and our skin looks drawn, pinched and grey; our immune system suffers, because it too becomes depressed. It is no coincidence that happy, optimistic people on the whole are sick less frequently, whereas depressed, pessimistic people become sick more often.

Simply remembering being in love, or remembering trauma, can release the same positive or destructive hormones and chemicals that were released during the event, because of our body's ability to respond equally to our thoughts as it does to actual events. In fact, events as such don't affect us, but it is the way we interpret an event and the meaning we choose to give to it that affects us.

After you have finished this programme you will be able to change the meaning and interpretation you have given to ageing.

Our psychological age is personal. In a matter of moments we can change how we feel. This affects our physiology – which is reflected in our body language and posture – and this in turn affects our organs. A good example of this is when we are feeling angry or upset and then something makes us laugh. Laughter is fantastic for reversing ageing. If you are feeling tired but hear some music that you love, it wakes you up, you dance around the room and your body language becomes very different from that of the tired person moments earlier, and you begin sending a different message to your organs.

In this programme I will show you what happens to your body when you take on the physiology of the old, the ill, the tired or depressed. Stooping, slumping, shuffling and hunching send the wrong kind of messages to your brain, whereas being active, vital, alive, joyful, dancing, singing and laughing send the right kind of messages to your brain and make the right kind of healing chemicals that you need to stay young.

Only our chronological age is fixed, and this should be ignored, because it is not important or even relevant. Our biological age is closely linked to our psychological age, so when we feel or act young or younger, our organs start to function and behave as young organs do. They literally begin to grow younger; however, when we feel and act old we begin to accelerate the ageing process, so our organs grow older.

This proves that how we age has much more to do with how we are as individuals than how we are as genetically, and how we are as individuals is something we can influence and change. We may not be able to change our genes, but we have vast powers to change ourselves; we have the power to succeed or fail at ageing, depending on how we choose to think, act, feel and react. We can all change, and we do change. Changing our thoughts and beliefs is a gift that only humans have. Animals don't have the same awareness. They cannot influence or change their thought processes. The major advantage and disadvantage in humans is that they have this power of choice. It is an advantage if you choose to become and stay younger, but it is a disadvantage if you choose to believe you cannot become younger and that ageing is beyond your control. There is so much that you can do to influence and direct how you age.

I have changed so much since studying human behaviour and human development that sometimes I can hardly recognise the person I was before. Nor can I believe that I ever used to think negative thoughts or hold pessimistic beliefs. I used to dread getting older, but now I look forward to every age because I know I can influence it. The changes you will make go much deeper than the fact that you can look and feel younger; you will also feel happier and more positive when you have a different concept of ageing that ensures you can age differently and more slowly than others who don't have this information to use.

It is so important to pay attention to our thoughts about ageing and the language we use. Our cells listen and react to our thoughts and words. If you say, 'I'm too old to do that', your mind and body will accept this literally. Believing you are too old will consequently cause you to feel and act older than you need to. In contrast, making a very simple change to your language and saying, 'I'm too tired to do that at the moment', will have a very different effect on your body.

With the understanding of these three ways of measuring age, if people say to you, 'You are getting too old to do that' or 'Well, its only to be expected at your age', you can quite honestly reply, 'Do you mean I'm too old chronologically, biologically or psychologically?'

We could look at an example of someone who has a chronological age of 50. Let's imagine this 50-year-old woman, who we will call Sara, exercises, eats healthy food and is predominantly happy and calm. She also practises yoga and she is able to relax by practising deep breathing, meditation or self-hypnosis. She is also a firm believer in the power of positive thinking and has good relationships.

Although Sara is chronologically 50, she could be biologically as young as 35. If we were to examine her lungs, heart, skin, hair, teeth, liver, kidneys, eyes and a variety of other organs, they would not all be 50. In fact they would vary greatly between 50 and 35. Her hair, nails and teeth would be younger than 50, her heart and lungs would be younger than 50 because she exercises, and let's assume she has protected her skin from the sun, so her skin is younger than 50 as well. She drinks a lot of water, so her kidneys are less than 50, and she is moderate with alcohol, so her liver is younger too. This woman is not fanatical, but she is taking control of how she ages in a very beneficial way. She has a good immune system, good circulation and good digestion, and she takes the time to breathe properly.

Now let us imagine a colleague of hers who is also chronologically 50 years old. Let's call her Jill. She doesn't exercise, her diet is unhealthy and she lives a very stressful life most of the time. Her job and family life are stressful. Perhaps she relaxes by smoking, having a drink or sunbathing.

Although Jill, like Sara, is chronologically 50, she could be biologically much older. If we were to examine her lungs, heart, skin, hair, teeth, liver, kidneys, eyes and other organs, they would not all be aged 50. In fact, they would vary greatly between less than 50 and, frequently, more than 50. Her nails and teeth could still be younger than 50, while her heart and lungs would be more than 50, because she smokes and does not exercise. And if we assume she has not protected her skin from the sun and has sunbathed frequently, her skin will be quite a lot older than 50. She drinks a lot of alcohol and not enough water, so her kidneys are above 50, as is her liver. Her immune system is not good because of her stress levels. Because she breathes in a shallow way, this, along with a poor diet, causes her to have poor digestion, which can disrupt all the systems of her body, thereby ageing her prematurely. This woman is not an extreme case, many people live this way, but she is failing to take control of how she ages and is ageing ahead of her chronological age.

As these examples show, your chronological age is not the same as your biological age, thus you can stop paying too much attention to that number. If you could live your life as if you had thrown away your birth certificate and didn't even know the date on it, how different would you be? There are some fascinating tribes where the people truly don't know their age, it is of no importance to them, and they are stronger and more powerful because they pay no attention at all to how old they are. The age you biologically are is of far more importance than the age you are in years, your chronological age.

Imagine that Sara feels young and believes that she is young: she laughs a lot, sings out loud and does young, fun things by playing tennis, going dancing and by listening to music that makes her feel alive, vital and joyful. She controls her mindset and has a positive attitude, and she seems to find the good in a situation. If she is stuck in traffic, she listens to some music or strikes up conversation, or she decides not to feel upset since the traffic is beyond her control. But her ability to choose what she thinks is hers to control and she does this successfully. She tells herself she is young and that she looks and feels young. She feels young psychologically and does not allow thoughts of her age to stop her doing things. Because Sara feels young psychologically, this has a very positive effect on her organs, which respond to the way she thinks and feels by ageing more slowly.

Jill, however, is very aware of getting older and allows thoughts of her age to influence what she does. She tells herself she is too old to do some things she might enjoy doing, she mentions her age far too much and thinks about it too much. It is the first thing she considers when new opportunities or invitations are presented to her. If her legs ache, she tells herself she's getting old without realising that this one thought is accelerating the ageing process. If she's invited to go on a trip she thinks she may be too old for the walking it could involve, or too old to mix with the others who perhaps are all younger. She tells herself she is too old and will look foolish if she takes up roller-blading or hot yoga. She turns down loud music telling herself she has grown out of that or is past the age for such things. If she is stuck in traffic she feels helpless and frustrated. If she forgets things, she tells herself it's all because of her age. Jill has not learned to control her mindset, and her attitude can be negative. This in turn has a detrimental effect on her organs, which respond to the way she thinks and feels by becoming older.

Don't be defined by your age

The fact that we all feel so many different ages at different times is proof that the number of years you have lived on the earth is not the age of your body or your mind or your emotions. Why, then, would you define yourself by the least important one – the one on your birth certificate?

When I am going on stage to give a seminar, I feel so excited. It's like going on a first date, and I feel about 20. When I am playing with children I feel about ten, but when I have to deal with a lot of responsibility or I don't like my daughter's new music, or if I have not had enough sleep, I can feel much older.

As you read the examples of Sara and Jill you might think, 'I lie in the sun, I drink and my diet isn't great, so what is the point of this programme? Hearing this is making me think I'm already biologically older than I should be.' The point is that the power of your mind and your ability to think different thoughts can override this. You may have heard of people who do unhealthy things yet remain young because they have a zest for life and an amazing attitude. You can do the same, because positive thinking has been proven to counteract even some negative habits. Keith Richards is not a role model for health, but his music and performing seem to have kept him young, which is why he is still performing at 70. When I went to the artist Molly Parkin's eightieth birthday party, she was in fabulous form, full of energy and happiness, and still going strong late into the night. Molly drank and smoked heavily right into her fifties, but she is ageing incredibly well because of her youthful attitude. If you are serious about becoming and remaining younger, obviously it's a good idea to make some lifestyle changes as well, and the final section of the book shows you some lifestyle changes that are easy to make, which will have an additional impact on the changes you are making.

This book is designed to give you factual information to illustrate that ageing, as we think we know it, is a misconception. You will do some easy tests to enable you to change your thoughts and beliefs. This first section will prepare you for change and to become younger. This section covers much of the groundwork necessary for you to change, not just mentally but physically too. You can actually change your biochemistry once you know how.

When you understand how your mind works and you learn how to communicate with your body so that it responds by slowing down ageing, you will know how to become and stay younger.

As you follow the step-by-step approach, you will easily understand what you should be doing, but please don't skip the exercises, as they are an important part of the book. If you make the time to follow the programme fully, you will still be reaping the benefits years from now.

You Can Be Younger is written in a way that will excite your imagination and your subconscious mind, making you ready for, and receptive to, changing both physically and mentally. The ability to excite the subconscious mind is a great asset in implementing positive permanent changes. Since most change is retroactive and cumulative, you may not notice immediate changes taking place, but they will be occurring. We don't notice headaches going, but we do notice when they have gone; we can lie in bed listening to a car alarm ringing and then later we will notice that it has stopped, but we didn't notice the moment when it actually stopped. These are examples of change being retroactive. People notice that they feel better only when they *are* better, but often they don't recognise it during the process itself. This applies to illness, grief and pain. We notice change mostly afterwards, as we look back on how we have changed, rather than as we are changing, so it can be hard to pinpoint the moment or time when the process of changing occurred.

An important point to remember as you go through this book is that you will be slowing down and reversing ageing inside your body, which will then effect visible outer changes. In the West we are very caught up with how we look on the outside, and although it is important to care about how we look, it is more important to work from inside our bodies than to concentrate on our outside appearance.

As you work through the book, if you expect to feel younger, to become younger and, of course, to look younger, you will, but you need also to be aware that the most important changes – the slowing down of the ageing of your organs – will be going on *within* your body. You may not see those results immediately, but they will be there. Some of the most important changes – those that can help you to maintain your hearing, eyesight and agility throughout life – may not show their impact for years. As you change your beliefs and the way you think, and as you alter in a positive way the images and thoughts you have about ageing, your mind will form a different concept of what ageing means. Because your mind controls your body, you will be able to change physically and mentally and stay younger.

To get the results you must commit yourself to doing the exercises as they are laid out for you. You only need a little time to let your mind accept each exercise. If you have the *conviction* that you can slow ageing, as well as the *desire* to go with this book and complete it, and the *belief* and the *faith* that it works, you have the ability within you to change your body – and this programme will give you that belief. If you persist in changing your thinking, you will succeed in becoming younger.

You may find it hard to believe now if you do not already have these opinions, but you will possess them when you have finished working through the book. This is not just a book to be read – it's a book to be used. Use the margins to write out notes, and write out the exercises as you follow the programme. Writing is very important; most successful people write out on paper what others keep in their minds. When you hold something in your mind it is a wish, a daydream, a fantasy, but when you write it out and commit it to paper it becomes more real because you can look at it and revise it. Also, writing things down enables the conscious mind to accept them and the subconscious mind to go to work to make them become a reality. Providing you make the changes required and allow these changes to become a part of your life you will be able to stay younger.

If you began an exercise programme that promised you a flatter stomach or firmer thighs, once you had achieved your goal you wouldn't quit the programme. You would stay on a maintenance programme to ensure you kept the results you had worked for. The same is true with this programme.

You can maintain the results you have achieved through using this book as long as you keep using the concept contained within it and continue to hear the messages it contains about ageing. It is worth re-reading parts of the book from time to time to remind yourself of the power of thought and the effect it has on you. It's also a good idea to re-read the things you have written and to review and recap them regularly.

When you are making mental changes and changing your thinking, you don't have to work hard, in fact you don't need to make a huge effort at all. It's not like doing physical exercises. Making mental changes is quite the opposite of the 'no pain no gain' theory. As long as you are open to the possibility of changing your thinking, you will be able to change it. Even thoughts that you may have held for years can be changed in seconds, as you will find. All it requires is that you absorb some new ideas, be open to change and be receptive to new possibilities. Our brains are already programmed to do this, almost as second nature, which is how we have evolved to progress and change over millions of years.

The best news is that some of the most simple changes described in the book are the ones that will have the most impact on slowing down the rate at which you age. You can consistently look and feel much younger while adding many more years to your life. You can look and feel vibrant, healthy and active into your eighties and beyond. You can live to enjoy more and more birthdays, yet be younger than many of your contemporaries, and you can help to change the view of ageing, which is based on a misconception. This is especially important to women, who are more habitually judged than men on their looks and on their youth. This is slowly changing, and you can do much to change it further, since before we can change any view collectively we first have to change it individually.

There are some wonderful women who have already changed our view of women as they age, women like Goldie Hawn,

Felicity Kendall, Helen Mirren, Lulu and Joanna Lumley, who have made the mid to late sixties sexy and youthful. Tina Turner appeared on the cover of *Vogue* looking amazing at the age of 73 while Jane Fonda brought out a new fitness DVD also at the age of 73, turning on its head the belief that we run out of energy and lose our looks and figure as we age. It's exciting to know that you can have the same impact on others as you change your own beliefs. We can help ensure that ageless men and women become the rule rather than the exception.

You are about to do something wonderful and powerful for you. You are going to change forever the way you see yourself, and you are going to change the way others see you. You are also going to change the way you feel, because you are ready now to begin following *You Can Be Younger*. As long as you use this programme correctly that is what you will be. This system really is foolproof – all you have to do is follow it.

Let's go.

Change Your Thoughts

'Imagination is more powerful than knowledge'

Albert Einstein (1879–1955)

In Step One you are going to change all your thoughts about ageing. You are going to learn how to *think and grow young*.

This is probably the most important lesson on how to slow down the ageing process: changing your thoughts. It is absolutely free and also the easiest for you to do, because you don't need to devote long periods of your time to it. When you begin to see how easy it is to change your thinking about ageing, you will find that you start changing your thinking about other areas of your life, with wonderful results.

All our thoughts have consequences. Every thought you are thinking, even now, has a consequence. A thought is a cause set in motion within us. When you become excited by this programme and believe what I am saying, you will already react differently from those who aren't sure, and those people will react differently from others who refuse to believe in this concept. In the area of ageing, our thoughts, beliefs and expectations about ageing will have a huge effect on how we age, because our body *must* mirror what is going on in our mind.

The mind acts to match our thoughts

The strongest and most powerful force in your mind is its need to act in ways that match your thinking. The strongest force in the human personality is the need to remain consistent with how we define ourselves. In other words, your body responds to the pictures you are making in your mind, and it constantly works to meet the picture. Your subconscious mind has little capacity to reason and it therefore believes whatever you tell it. The subconscious mind has no sense of humour, so let's imagine that it's your birthday and you see an outfit you want to buy. You try it on, you look in the mirror and say:

'I look ancient in this.'

Perhaps you are saying it as a joke just to yourself about getting older, perhaps you are laughing with your friends or perhaps you are hoping one of them will reassure you and say you look great. They probably will, but it's too late, your mind is already accepting what you say, quite literally, because that is what it is set up and designed to do. It cannot do anything else. Now your mind has to make a picture of the thought 'ancient', which it will probably see as something very old and fragile, and not at all the image you want for yourself. Your mind then has to work so that you match that picture and physically feel in a way that mirrors the picture of the word 'ancient'.

I know that you can't possibly want to see yourself as ancient, so you must stop thinking those thoughts and using those words.

One of my friends sent out invitations to her birthday party and told everyone that she was becoming an antique. It was a very funny invitation, except that as her mind literally believes she is becoming an antique it now *has* to make her respond that way. So how does the mind see an antique? It sees it as very old and very fragile. Oh well, at least an antique has some value and can be priceless, but you are not an antique, so don't use that word if you want to stay young. Remember all those funny birthday cards with all the wit about becoming past it, the ones that show two prunes in a bowl and say that you know you are getting old when your breasts look like this. Yes, they are funny, and I am not suggesting you lose your sense of humour. In fact, laughing is one of the best medicines in the world, and it makes you feel young, so laugh at the jokes, but do not even for a moment believe what they say, and do not make jokes about ageing and relate them to yourself. Most people joke about getting old because they are scared and nervous of the prospect of ageing, but after this programme you can allay the fear and dread of ageing, so you don't need to joke about it.

Replacing a negative thought with a positive one

Many of you hearing me talk about changing your thoughts will think, 'But how do I stop thinking a thought, since it is instant?' It will get easier, I promise, and you can assist this by dismissing every negative thought you have about ageing and replacing it with a new, constructive one instead. Your thoughts belong to you. Why would you keep them if you don't want them and don't want to believe them? But your thoughts are also yours to change.

What we see we become, and what we think about all the time we become, so think about being younger and you will be younger. It sounds almost too simple doesn't it? But it works. The power of thought may be simple, but thoughts themselves are enormously powerful and effective. You cannot have any thoughts and feelings without them being expressed in your body. You can't feel sad or happy, hot or tired, miserable or delighted, without those feelings being expressed in your body. When you are feeling old, those feelings also have to be expressed in your body, which is why I never use the word 'old' but instead I tell myself I am feeling tired or stressed, because to the body these are temporary feelings, but old is permanent.

Thoughts create images that become reality

We can all take charge of programming our minds, because the way we feel from one moment to the next is a result of only two things: the pictures we make in our head and the words we are using. The mind especially responds to thoughts, words and images that are symbolic. I know you are thinking, 'Why should that be?' and 'How can that happen?', so here's an example: if you describe your favourite food to someone, you will already start to make saliva and digestive enzymes and can even start to feel physically hungry, because your mind is responding to the words and pictures you are making.

The good news is that you are able to choose the pictures you make in your mind, to choose what you say, think and feel about ageing. Through your power of choice, through your ability to choose your thoughts and beliefs about ageing you can succeed in becoming and remaining younger at every stage of your life.

Even the habit of thought precedes the habit of action, so if you believe you have to smoke to concentrate, or you need to drink to relax, that belief will eventually become more powerful than the habit itself. This is why when changing habits you must also change the *beliefs* related to the habits, thus ensuring that you don't return to them.

If you go to exercise classes to retain a youthful figure and muscle tone, or if you take antioxidants to fight ageing, but you doubt either the exercise or the antioxidants' ability to work, or if you believe that ageing is inevitable regardless, these thoughts can, and will, work against all the work you are doing. In contrast, if you believe that you will influence how you age, and you decide to change your thinking, and then you change your habits of thought and also change your habits of action to adopt a healthier lifestyle with improved nutrition, you can expect to achieve wonderful results that will stay with you throughout your life.

Because of our mind's ability to believe and accept without

question, to accept as an absolute fact all our thoughts and dialogue, including the internal dialogue or self-talk that goes on inside our heads, it follows that if you constantly tell yourself that you are getting old you will become that way. The reverse is also true: if you keep telling yourself you are remaining youthful you will remain that way instead.

The mistake of labelling actions as caused by age

If you tell yourself you are forgetful or clumsy, you will become that way at any age. Even telling this to young children can cause them to act and become clumsy and forgetful. If you tell yourself you are forgetful because you are getting older, you will begin to identify and act in ways that match that thinking. If you decide you may be showing early signs of Alzheimer's or dementia, you must abandon that thought immediately. Don't even entertain the idea or put words or pictures relating to it in your mind. It is OK to forget things – children are always forgetting their homework, leaving their coat at school or their lunch box at their friend's house, but we don't say, 'You are so forgetful. It must be your age.'

At every age we can return from the shop having forgotten something, but as soon as we hit 40 we seem to blame it on our age. So what was the reason when you were 16 or 24 and you forgot? You didn't blame it on your age then, you just forgot.

I spent one New Year in Greece with my friends and our children, and we all stayed up extremely late. The next day one of my friends must have said at least ten times, 'I'm too old for late nights now, I feel dreadful. I can't stay up late like I used to,' adding, 'I'm so cranky because I really need my sleep at my age.' I pointed out to her that our children were also tired and even more cranky than we were, because they also needed their sleep, but we weren't saying 'they are too old for late nights'; instead we said, 'They didn't have enough sleep, they stayed up too late so they are not feeling their best, but tomorrow they will be back to normal.'

The self-fulfilling prophecy of inherited conditions

Some doctors believe that when migraines, depression or period pains run in families it is because the mind has accepted this as inevitable and the body acts accordingly. So often when working with clients they tell me things like, 'Everyone in my family has allergies', 'All the women in my family have had problems conceiving', 'My mother suffered terribly with sinus pain and I'm just like her', and so on, without being aware of how they are identifying with the symptom. Of course, there are illnesses that are hereditary, but it is very important not to identify with something you don't want, especially in the area of our health and ageing. When talking about children, if you say, 'He has a temper just like his father' or 'She has problems spelling just like me' or 'He has a nervous rash like his grandfather', it projects that into their identity, which is exactly what you don't want.

As you will see later, identity beliefs affect everything we do and are extremely powerful. The body *must* match what is going on in the mind – it is never the other way around. The mind *won't* match what is going on in the body, because thought always has to come first and every thought eventually becomes expressed in the body or through the body.

Ageing has become an expectation that we live up to in our minds *and then* in our bodies. The way you expect to age, and the beliefs you hold about ageing, are having an enormous effect on how you are ageing *right now*. It has been said that the body you have today is a result of the thoughts about ageing you were thinking ten years ago, and the body you will have in ten years' time will be a result of the thoughts about ageing you are thinking now.

Finding a new dialogue

That idea can be scary or quite reassuring, depending on the thoughts you are having, but your thoughts are absolutely yours to change, and changing them gets easy once you begin. We are constantly thinking thoughts and holding a dialogue with ourselves about mundane daily things, saying things like, 'I must remember to charge my phone', 'I'm hungry', 'What time is it?', 'Where did I put my keys?' and so on. This programme really isn't going to ask you to do anything that you don't already do. What it will do is train you to do all these things in a much better way so that you are running your mind rather than your mind running you.

Your thoughts about ageing are affecting your body this very second. The body mimics the mind's thoughts. Every thought we have creates a physical reaction in the body and an emotional response, but our thoughts and beliefs are not fixed and are ours to change. Thinking young thoughts, telling yourself your cells are young, causes them to respond, to act and behave as young cells do. Our cells listen and respond to our thinking, so if you come in from a long or tiring day having planned to go out that evening and think to yourself or say to anyone listening, 'I'm too old to go out in the evenings, I can't cope with late nights anymore', your mind and body will accept this literally and believe that you are indeed too old. It will cause you to feel and act older.

In contrast, making a very simple change to your thoughts and thinking, 'I'm too tired to go out this evening' will have a very different effect on your body, because it is a temporary rather than a permanent feeling and belief. It does not mean that you will be too tired tomorrow.

It isn't always automatic to change our thinking. Sometimes we have to keep at it because we have been so conditioned to believe ageing is unavoidable. Even I, who of all people should know better, still catch myself blaming age occasionally. I came out of the gym recently, my knee twinged and my instant thought was that my knees are getting older. Our thoughts are so instant, it is easy to feel that they are running us, but we must think more consciously about it:

- Where did that belief come from?
- Who put it there?
- Why am I choosing to believe this?

As I had that thought about my knee, I had to dismiss it immediately and then replace it with another thought by reminding myself that joints can ache or twinge at any age. My knee could be twingeing from not exercising it properly and it has nothing to do with my age.

We can use the power of the mind to stay youthful, active and healthy, so we are young, whatever our years. You can choose to believe that youth is energy, flexibility and attitude, to know that if you think old thoughts and use ageing language you will become old, so make doing the opposite a lifelong habit. You will have to work at this initially, but it will become second nature after a while and will be so worth it.

Everything we do and everything we want is because of how it makes us feel. Think of anything right now that you want, and I bet you want it because of the way it will make you feel. We want money, status and youth, because we believe they will make us feel better. Changing your thoughts about how you are going to age will undoubtedly cause you to feel better physically, mentally and emotionally.

I am going to show you throughout this book that our body doesn't age in the way we have been led to believe, and since the mind can be ageless, it makes all the beliefs and negative expectations we have learned and falsely held to be true about ageing meaningless and pointless. You are unique, and you are certainly ageing uniquely and according to your own timetable, but you have a great capacity to influence this in a positive way. Because we all age uniquely, we must change forever these self-limiting beliefs about ageing that only exist in our imagination. Our thoughts and beliefs are absolutely ours to change. We can always control our thoughts and what things mean, and then anything is possible.

We can also let go of long-held thoughts

Just because we have held something to be true for a number of years it is not a good enough reason to hold on to it any longer. You used to believe in Father Christmas once, but you then changed your beliefs as you acquired new information. My daughter used to believe that fairies lived at the bottom of our garden, and she was convinced she had seen the Easter bunny, but it is easy and automatic to give up these beliefs once we acquire new information. When children suddenly decided that they don't believe in Father Christmas anymore it's because they are at an age where they are changing and re-evaluating their beliefs all the time as they come across new information. You are doing the same thing as you read this book.

The human nervous system is the only nervous system aware of ageing. Animals have no such awareness and they can't do anything to slow down ageing, but we can. We can use that same awareness to influence our cells and to slow down ageing. We must never despair of, or dread, growing old, as that thought can make us age more quickly. We are only ever as old as we think we are, since our cells process our thoughts and we eventually become our beliefs of age and ageing. It is the same if we believe that we are forgetful, clumsy or unlovable. We move towards the thoughts and beliefs we hold until we eventually become a living, walking, talking, expression of them. A belief or feeling that we are unlovable is the common denominator of most emotional problems in the Western world, so if you think that only youth is desirable – an image that advertisers sell to us relentlessly – if you think that only youth is loveable, it is not surprising that you may dread ageing.

Ageing in the modern world

Today, ageing is new and different from the past. It has been called the New Old Age simply because old age now for many people is a positive, healthy and enjoyable time of life. I think it would be more enjoyable still if the term 'old age' was used less frequently and something with a more positive image was used instead. The New Old Age is better; 'sageing' might be better than 'ageing'.

Ageing no longer needs to be feared as a time when we inevitably deteriorate or become sedentary and fragile. It can be quite different, and already is for many of us. Judi Dench, Maggie Smith, Mary Berry and even Bruce Forsyth are inspiring examples of older people who are far from fragile or sedentary. The power of thought alone can change the physical body and affect our mental health and our immune system. What we think is possible affects our body. People can actually appear to be 'getting drunk' on alcohol-free beverages because they think they are potent; others feel their symptoms of illness improve on placebo medication.

The power of suggestion

This thought process can become even stronger when it occurs in groups; for example, mass sickness can occur on airlines or at functions when people wrongly believe they have been infected or exposed to the offending bacteria. At the Monterey Park football stadium in Los Angeles, several people became ill with symptoms of food poisoning during a game. The onsite doctor treating them, on discovering that they had all drunk Coca-Cola from the vending machines at the stadium, decided that fermentation or contamination could have taken place within the vending machines. Eager that no one else would be put at risk, he organised an announcement requesting that no one drink from the machines, because of the illness, and described the symptoms over the air. Almost at once the stadium became a sea of retching and fainting, including people who had not drunk anything from the suspected machines. Five ambulances were carrying people back and forth between the hospital and the stadium before it was discovered that the vending machines were safe and the illness of the first group was unrelated. Eventually, normality was restored.

You can find many examples of the power of thought suggestion and beliefs. Thoughts have very direct consequences. At Massachusetts General Hospital, anaesthesiologist Dr Henry Beecher found that 30 per cent of a drug's or a doctor's success is due to the patient's expectation of a desired outcome, or the 'placebo effect'.[4] The American Society of Psychosomatic Medicine, founded in 1955, further explored the placebo effect. Today, drug companies routinely discard over 30 per cent of drug test results, because if a person believes a drug to be effective, it can have more effect on him or her than the drug itself. This is why many repeat drug prescriptions are placebos and why whenever a drug is tested it must also be tested on a control group who think they are receiving the same drug but are in fact receiving a placebo.

Illness and its link to our belief system

Our beliefs about the drugs and medicines we take can be even more significant in our recovery than the pharmaceutical components of the drugs themselves. Dr Beecher became famous for carrying out extensive research and numerous studies which concluded that while we may believe a particular drug has healed or cured us, in fact it was our belief system that was the real healing force. In his 1955 paper 'The powerful placebo', Dr Beecher went on record stating, 'A drug's usefulness is a direct result of not only the chemical properties of the drug, but also the patient's belief in the usefulness and effectiveness of the drug.' This can have fascinating results. In the US, when a new drug formulated to re-grow hair was tested, the group given placebo pills re-grew hair, despite many of them having been bald for years. In another test in the UK, 30 per cent of a group who believed they were receiving a new form of chemotherapy lost all their hair purely because they expected to, but unbeknownst to them they were receiving placebos.[5]

OUR THOUGHTS ARE INTRICATELY CONNECTED TO OUR BODY

Our brain converts our expectations into chemical realities. Thoughts are things, and thoughts always have an effect on our bodies. Thinking about hunger, sex or tiredness will cause us to generate feelings and physical reactions that are linked to our thinking. Reading books that describe immense cold can make us shiver and grow goose bumps, and watching a scary or emotional film can generate feelings of fear or emotion within ourselves that seem quite real.

Of course, advertising companies know all about this and use it to their advantage. Images of food can cause us to feel hungry, whereas images of drinks make us thirsty. Even very young chil-dren have been proven to respond to adverts. In fact, the children's television programme *Sesame Street* used the same suc-cessful format of short bursts of message, sound and colour that are used to make adverts, as it maximises children's ability to respond.

We see more examples of the power of thought in telepathy and in people who appear to have unusual powers, such as faith healers and mind readers. Often, just being around someone we perceive as powerful, or being in a place such as Lourdes that has a powerful effect on the belief system, is enough for us to see results, regardless of what is real and what is imagined.

Years ago, a client came to see me because he wanted to stop drinking. He sat on the other side of my desk while I asked him some questions. Suddenly he looked at me and said, 'I can't answer any more questions, this hypnosis is too powerful,' and he then slumped back in his chair, closed his eyes and went into a trance purely because he expected to. In fact I had not hypnotised him. As he was already responding to his own power of thought, I used the situation to convince his subconscious that he would not drink again and to uncover the causes of drinking and the beliefs that made him drink too much. He called me some weeks later to tell me how thrilled he was to not even want to drink any-more, and to this day I still have clients who come in to see me who were referred to me by this man. They always tell me that he is a major fan of hypnosis and me, since I had such a powerful effect on him. I didn't ever have the heart to tell him that I did very little. It was his own belief system that stopped him drinking.

Further examples of this are apparent from other cultures where people may believe they have been cursed and who then begin to develop symptoms linked to their beliefs, sometimes even causing deaths. In Africa, this is known as shaking or pointing the bone. If the witch doctor shakes the bone the person this is directed to will expect to get ill and perhaps die. In cases where medical intervention has taken place to cure the resulting illness or symptoms, that sometimes isn't enough, because the medication cannot always overcome that person's belief system which is convinced that they are cursed and dying.

The belief system is the stronger force and has more power than anything else. People who have moved from the West to Haiti, for example, and who had hitherto scorned the belief in voodoo, magic and other similar traditions, often begin to change their views about it because these beliefs are all around them. They become somewhat influenced by the pervasive effect it has on them.

Other common examples of the power of thought occur with the symptoms of phantom pregnancies and psychosomatic ill-nesses. In the case of phantom pregnancies the thought of pregnancy is so strong that it generates the physical symptoms of pregnancy in the body.

The power of the mind put to the test

A thought is a cause set in motion within us. The Bible states, 'As a man thinketh he becometh.'

Dr Ellen Langer, a psychologist at Harvard Medical School, put this to the test in 1979, when she took a group of men, all over 75 years old, to a retreat in the country for seven days. Prior to leaving, the group was put through a series of tests to establish each person's biological age. Among other things, they were tested for hearing, vision, grip, finger length, muscle mass, bone density, perception, physical strength, blood, hormones, and so on. The retreat had been designed to recreate the year 1959, and the participants even wore badges with pictures of themselves from 20 years previously. They watched films, sitcoms and newsreels, and listened to music from the 1950s. All the magazines and newspapers were from the 1950s, and the participants were not allowed to bring with them anything from a later date.

The group then purposefully pretended it was 20 years earlier. The conversation and everything else going on around them was deliberately engineered to enable and encourage each man to act as he had when he was 55 rather than 75. Meanwhile, a control group went to the same retreat but did not have to pretend or live in the artificially back-dated environment.

By willingly participating in and living this experiment, the main participants were subconsciously tricking themselves – and consequently their cells – to believe they were younger. During the seven days, and at the end, they were put through the same tests again. All had reversed their biological age by a minimum of seven years. Some had reversed their age by over ten years. By contrast, the control group improved very marginally in a few areas but declined in others.

In 2010, the BBC recruited Dr Langer to repeat the programme with a group of British celebrities. Those taking part included the actresses Liz Smith (88 years old), Sylvia Syms (76), cricket umpire Dickie Bird (77), dancer Lionel Blair (77) and journalist Derek Jameson (80). Just as in the 1979 experiment, the group stayed in a large country house that had been fitted with furnishings and kitchen and electrical appliances that would have been seen in 1975. The newspapers and television programmes available to them were also from 1975, and each person's bedroom was decorated to look as much like it would have in the 1970s, complete with personal mementoes from the time.

The experiment started off like the earlier US one, and the participants had to take care of themselves right from the beginning. When they arrived at the house where they would be staying for a week, they had to carry their own bags upstairs. Liz Smith was the only one who didn't do it, as she had been assigned to a bedroom on the ground floor. She was unable to walk more than a few steps without the aid of two sticks and had to use a wheelchair when going outside. Within days, each of the celebrities had considerably improved. Liz Smith managed to walk around the kitchen with just one stick. She even managed a bit of dancing! Sylvia Syms ran around the garden with two dogs, with youthful gusto. They all showed great improvements just halfway through the week.

Then some professional carers came in and offered to do everything for the participants. Some agreed and quickly reverted to their old selves. When the carers left again, in the afternoon, things soon got back on track. After the help left, Lionel Blair said it had made him feel much older. Liz Smith agreed. Sylvia Syms had steadfastly refused any help.

By the end of the seven days, it was clear that all the participants were much better at doing various things than they had been just one week earlier. They all had better balance, flexibility, upper and lower body strength, and a more positive outlook on life. Liz Smith was able to walk more than 140 paces across the garden, with only one stick. In the final physical examination, she was able to stand on one leg without holding on to anything. She even went out dancing when she returned home. Lionel Blair danced with a tap-dancing group and looked very agile, matching the movements and speed of the men who were about one-third his age. Sylvia Syms is now helping with a charity that assists older people. She said that when she first started on the experiment, she was in considerable pain all the time from back injuries, and she had no energy. She was running about by the end of the exercise and said that she had no back pain and had more energy.

Derek Jameson could hardly get up the stairs at the beginning, but halfway through he was doing step-ups on a low step. At the start, he couldn't even put his own socks on, so bad was his flexibility, but by the end, he could do it. Dickie Bird felt as if he had a new lease of life. His strength, memory and agility improved. Since suffering a stroke, he had been living without much contact with other people and had lost a lot of confidence, but he was determined to take part in life again. It was particularly satisfying to see him laughing and enjoying himself, as since retirement he had become a self-confessed recluse. As Jameson was packing to go home at the end of the week, he explained what had happened to make them all feel so much younger. He said that he'd forgotten that he was 80 and that he had slipped back into the 1970s and lived in that world of 35 years earlier.

These experiments proved that what you believe is so important in determining how you age, and what happens if you think you are too old. If you think and act old, you may grow old prematurely, whereas if you think and act younger, you can remain younger physically, mentally and biologically.

WORD ASSOCIATIONS

In another BBC television programme, members of the public were asked to make sentences out of words to test their language proficiency. The first group was given words that are usually associated with old age, such as 'obedient', 'accepting', 'wise', 'courteous', 'alone', 'sentimental' and 'careful'. The group was filmed entering the building, and again after the test, as they left the room and walked along a corridor. Most of them walked more slowly (some 10 or 20 per cent slower), as if using words associated with old age had made them behave older.

A second group participated in the same test but used words that are usually associated with youth, such as 'ambition', 'freedom', 'attractive', 'fashion' and 'passion'. Most of them walked more quickly afterwards – as much as 10 or 15 per cent faster.

THE BRAIN CAN RISE TO A NEW CHALLENGE

In another experiment, people were told they were going to be tested to see if they would be good fighter pilots. They wore pilot overalls and were tested in a flight simulator for a Harrier jump jet. Their eyesight was tested before and afterwards. Most of them could read more letters on the eye chart after the experiment. Their eyes hadn't improved, but it is thought that their brains were working harder – as if they were still trying to be like fighter pilots. Fighter pilots need excellent vision, so their brains were trying to give them that.

Become younger by changing your focus and language

Changing our thinking and our behaviour has a physical effect on the ageing of our minds and bodies. These tests proved that we can become biologically seven years younger, and more, in just seven days, and we can learn a lot from them.

You can become biologically and physically younger by changing your beliefs and recreating your notion of who you are and what you associate with ageing. Changing your focus and your language can slow down the way you age and has been proven to reverse it.

As we have seen, thoughts always affect the skin, which is why it boasts a rosy glow when we are in love or feeling happy and good about ourselves, but it looks grey or drawn when we are grieving or deeply unhappy. Scientific tests have shown that people who were anxious began to look older within just a few months, but when they resolved the cause of their anxiety they began to reverse this premature ageing and returned to looking younger even more rapidly. Begin now to change your thoughts about what ageing is and what your age means. Delete all negative words connected to ageing from your vocabulary. If, for example, you look in the mirror and think, 'My skin looks old', decide instead that your skin looks tired or dehydrated. Although ageing does happen to skin, your skin also has wonderful rejuvenating abilities. By changing your thinking you can absolutely change your body. Beliefs create biology, and the mind is the most powerful healing force there is.

USE PICTURES TO CREATE YOUTHFUL REMINDERS

You could create a kind of Ellen Langer retreat in your home, in just one corner of one room. Using a notice board, pin up photos of you at your most agile and vital, and include some pictures of yourself as a child. Look especially for pictures where you look carefree and spontaneous. You could write out some lines from poems or words from your favourite songs about how youth is just a state of mind.

A very inspiring method is to make a mood board or collage by cutting out pictures that symbolise or represent the kind of youthfulness you plan to achieve. Include in this collage role models – people who are similar to your age but look and act younger – and find pictures from magazines of older people skiing or practising yoga, and include them as well. Stick onto the mood board the words or poems that inspire you to be young, find some quotes that you like, or copy some from this book onto your mood board. You could also write or stick onto the mood board the affirmations and goals and your personal programme for becoming younger that you will be learning later on in this book.

Boost your immune system

Your thoughts will even affect your immune system. By changing the way you think and by changing your beliefs and your language, plus making some modifications in the way you eat, sleep and behave, you can greatly influence how you age at every stage of your life. It all starts with adjusting how you think – you can add many full and youthful years to your life.

Most people don't want to live to be 100 if their quality of life is awful, but we can live long lives and stay much younger and healthier. We can continue to look and feel 5, 10 and eventually even 15 years younger than we are by changing our thinking and making the changes outlined in this book.

Just knowing that life expectancy is rapidly increasing means that middle age, which used to be from our thirties onwards, now doesn't even need to begin until we are in our fifties. Stop and think about that for a moment: middle age is being pushed further and further away. Doesn't just knowing that make you feel younger already? If you want to change anything about your body, health, weight or relationships, first you must change your thinking. Everything that is going on in your body, including ageing, has to start with the mind. For any area of your life that you want to change or control you must begin by transforming your thoughts:

- Your thoughts control your feelings.
- Your feelings control your actions.
- Your actions control events.

If you think you hate flying or if you suffer with travel sickness, that will, of course, control how you feel about getting on an aeroplane. That, in turn, will probably cause you to avoid the action of flying and make events around you different from those of someone who loves to fly. This thought will influence the type of holidays you take and possibly even the type of job you choose.

TAKE CONTROL

It is essential that you take control of how you age. In life, so many things appear to be out of our control. In fact, the only real control we have over events is what we choose to think of them and what we decide something means. We are ageing differently and better than ever before, so thinking good thoughts about ageing and interpreting ageing differently, as well as believing that we can get older without getting old, and that we can look, feel and become younger, will have an immediate and ultimately visible and lasting effect on our bodies.

Women frequently get to their thirties and then begin a lifelong and destructive habit of saying, 'I'm too old to wear that now' or 'I'm too old to go there any longer' or 'I'm too old for that.' Men usually start reacting in this way later on. I recently had a client who asked me if I thought it was OK for him to still wear Levi's because he felt he was becoming too old to wear them – and he was 35. Around us we hear others saying, 'Act your age' or 'You shouldn't be doing that at your age' or 'Aren't you a little old to be doing that?' No one would say that to Tina Turner, who was happier and more attractive in her fifties than she was in her thirties, and now at 74 is still an exuberant and beautiful woman who recently got married. She is regarded as an exception, but she is not an exception; she is a great example of how changing our thinking changes our reality.

How do we know that Tina Turner is not an example of how normal ageing could look and that we are the exceptions? No one can say for sure that this could not be a possibility.

THE BENEFITS OF HAPPINESS

Happiness has a profound effect upon your body. Recent tests showed that when newly in-love couples were given a small amount of poison, their bodies did not react to it at all. When a much smaller amount of the same poison was given to people who were sad, unhappy and alone, they reacted immediately and became unwell.

When we are in love, we are constantly being told by our partner, 'You're amazing, you're so great, I love you, I adore you.' Hearing these words has an effect on our immune system, and it becomes stronger. Hearing negative words has the opposite effect, and our immune system becomes weaker.

YOUR IMAGINATION CAN BOOST YOUR IMMUNE SYSTEM

At the Rainbow Children's Hospital in Cleveland, a group of children were shown a puppet show. One puppet represented a germ and the other puppet was the immune system. The immune system puppet, which was made to look like a policeman, fought the germ and defeated it. The children were then asked to close their eyes and imagine the puppets in their bodies, with lots of immune system puppets killing all the germs. This lasted for only a few minutes, and then saliva samples were taken from the children. The results of the saliva samples showed that their immunoglobulin levels had increased significantly. (Immunoglobulin is a protein released by the body when it's under attack from infection.) The children's immune systems had responded as if they were fighting a real infection, as if a virus was actually present, and they were stronger as a result, even though the virus existed only in their imaginations.

Scientists have irrefutable evidence that we can all boost our immune systems just by thinking about them in a particular way. You can boost your health and slow down ageing just by thinking of it in a more positive way.

I am now going to show you how every thought has a physical effect and an emotional response within your body. I would like you to do a few very simple and perfectly safe exercises to demonstrate the amazing physical powers of thought so that you can feel it and experience it for yourself rather than just reading about it.

Exercise 1: The pull of a magnet

1   Stand up with your feet slightly apart. Close your eyes and begin to imagine that just behind you there is a huge magnet, pulling you and rocking you backwards. Really focus on the magnet. See it as a huge traditional U-shaped magnet with the red paint on the curve, just behind your shoulder blades.

2   You will almost immediately feel yourself swaying and rocking, and tipping backwards. You might even notice that your knees lock and your toes lift off the floor.

3   Now imagine the magnet has moved to just under your chin and is pulling you forwards. Again, as you think about the magnet pulling you forwards, your own power of thought will cause you to rock and sway forwards and to move off your heels.

▶

4   Now imagine the magnet has moved to your right
    shoulder and notice your body swaying in that
    direction so that your hips and shoulder pull to the
    right; then imagine it moving to the left. The more you
    focus on the magnet, the stronger the pull will
    become. Just notice it happening.

If you prefer, you can close your eyes and ask a friend to
describe a magnet behind you, then in front of you, and
then at either side of your shoulder, or ask someone to
read this exercise to you.
    Of course, there is no magnet there, but you are
beginning to see and feel for yourself your mind's ability
to accept whatever you tell it, whether it's based on fact
or fiction. As your mind accepts the thought of the
magnet, it then works to have you react to it, even
though it exists only in your imagination.

The same is true with every thought that you have. If you think of
remaining young in looks and actions, your mind has to accept
that and work on it. Even more importantly, your cells and your
immune system will react to the thought. If you think of being
old, the same thing happens, so one thought can generate positive
reactions within the body and another thought can generate negative reactions. Whether these thoughts are based on fact or
fiction is irrelevant to the mind, because it cannot tell the difference. Here is another safe and simple exercise to prove to you that
thought really is extremely powerful. You can do this while sitting
or standing.

Exercise 2: A heavy bucket and a light balloon

1   Close your eyes. Stretch both hands out in front of you at shoulder height, and close both hands as if you are holding reins or a bar in each hand.

2   Now begin to imagine that in your left hand you are holding an enormous red fire bucket filled with extremely heavy, wet sand. Feel the weight of that bucket in your fingers. Feel the weight moving up to your wrist, your elbow, and now your shoulder. Feel it getting heavier and heavier by the second, and notice that your arm is being pulled down by the weight of the bucket. The more you focus on the bucket, on its colour, size and contents, the heavier your arm is becoming, and the more it is being drawn downwards.

3   As your left arm continues moving downwards, imagine that you are holding in your right hand the biggest helium-filled balloon. See the balloon's colour as bright blue. See it as almost bigger than you are. Feel the string in your hand. As helium is lighter than air, and because this balloon is firmly held in your right hand, you will notice that your right arm is moving upwards, travelling up higher and higher, becoming lighter and lighter, almost floating upwards of its own accord.

4   As you think about the balloon and bucket, notice the difference in your arms. One is heavy, one is light; one is moving up, the other is moving down. The cause of this is your thought process.

You may prefer to memorise this or to have someone read this exercise to you while you keep your eyes shut.

The point once again is to show you how easy it is to influence your mind and to prove to you that thoughts have a very real effect on our bodies.

Keep focused for maximum benefits

Because the strongest force in the mind is its need to make us act in ways that match our thinking, it is vital to change any negative thoughts, beliefs and expectations connected to ageing, so you must:

> Focus on how you want to be,
> never on how you don't want to be.

In other words:

> Keep your mind on what you want
> and off what you don't want.

Therefore, regarding ageing and in all areas of life:

- Focus only on what you want to move towards and accomplish.
- Never focus on the opposite, as this is what you want to move away from.

This becomes easier as you find the flip side of every negative thought and use that instead. Remember:

- Whatever we focus on we move towards.
- Whatever we focus on we experience and feel.
- Whatever we focus on we get more of, and it becomes more real to us.

If you focus on having an injection, or the pressure in your ears during a flight descent, you can make it painful, even very painful, but if you focus on something else you may not even notice the sensations.

Now we are ready to do some written exercises, so you will need a notebook.

Exercise 3: Recognise your negative thoughts

1   In your notebook write out all your thoughts about ageing that are related to you. Write out every negative thought that you have been led to believe about ageing on one page, and then write out new and more appropriate thoughts on the opposite page.

2   Keep writing until you have run out of thoughts, but don't be surprised if more come to you later. As they do, write them out in your book.

The reason I want you to write out negative thoughts is because often we are not even aware of our thoughts. We hold them, we act on them, but we don't confront them or look at them or think, 'Is this relevant to me? Has it ever been relevant to me?' We revamp our wardrobes and update our homes, yet we fail to update our thinking. Before we can change our thinking we need to identify and discover our thoughts. This section will allow you to become more and more aware of your thoughts in order to update them and to review and revise them.

▶

Take some time to uncover your thoughts about how you are ageing. Become more and more aware of how you think. Take as much time as you need. Find and root out any negative thoughts, then change them or eliminate them. As you start writing, your thoughts will begin to flow from you. Don't stop to analyse them, but just keep on writing. It doesn't matter whether you write out reams of thoughts or just a few, as long as they are your thoughts. The most important thing is to write out what you think about ageing and what your point of view about ageing is.

Start changing your thinking now

This book will allow you to use the new knowledge and facts within it to stop your old negative thinking, and in its place you will have new and powerful positive thoughts that you really believe in and which can affect how you age in the most wonderful way. You can use your mind to tell yourself that you are staying young instead of rationalising why you have to get old.

Here are some examples to give you an idea and to get you started on the process of changing your thinking.

EXAMPLES OF NEGATIVE THINKING

You may have said some of these things yourself:

- I noticed the skin on my legs was dry and thought to myself that it was an inevitable part of ageing.

- I forgot to buy some essential items while I was in the supermarket and thought I must be getting old and forgetful.
- I couldn't seem to thread a needle, so I asked my son to do it and said, 'My eyesight is not as good as it was. It must be my age.'
- I had a late night and felt tired the next day and now I remember how often I have told my partner, 'I can't stay up late like I used to', 'I'm getting too old for late nights', 'I need my sleep at my age', 'I can't go to late-night parties anymore', and so on.
- While out shopping I looked at the fashions and decided I was too old to wear those clothes anymore, so I chose safe, older clothes even though I know they make me feel and look older than I need to.
- I am now aware of how often I think I shouldn't really do that or wear this at my age.

EXAMPLES OF POSITIVE THINKING

Here are a few new thoughts to replace the negative ones:

- I will moisturise my skin daily, drink more water and keep my skin hydrated.
- Even when I was 20 I forgot things. My memory is great, and the odd slip up has nothing to do with my age.
- My eyesight is fine, and if I don't see something well I will blame the light or perhaps being tired, but I will never attribute it to my age. After all, at my grandmother's sewing circle she and her friends produce the most intricate stitching, so they must have good eyesight and they are all 80 years plus.
- I can stay up late and have fun. It doesn't matter if I feel tired

the next day. My children are tired all the next day if they stay up late and I never say they are getting too old for late nights since they are all under ten years old.

- I can adapt fashions and look stylish at any age. Dressing appropriately has more to do with my figure than my age. I can wear modern fashions and bright colours if I choose to.
- I feel and look young. I believe I am young, so anything I want to do or wear suits me.

Summary – Step One

So let's recap everything you have learned so far.

- You have learned the absolute power of thoughts and how to change your thinking.
- You now know that thoughts are things and that every single thought you have has a physical effect on your body and an emotional effect on your mind. All of your thoughts have consequences. Your healthy thoughts have healthy consequences, whereas negative thoughts will eventually have negative consequences.
- All thoughts in the mind have to produce responses in the body, so by applying the techniques in this book and learning to accept only positive thoughts, ideas and beliefs about ageing you can programme your body to grow younger.
- You have also learned that your thoughts are yours to change, to update, to review and remove as they cease to be appropriate to you.
- You have learned how and why ageing cannot be defined and how you can rethink ageing in a positive way.
- You have learned how our modern lifespan is changing greatly.

- By doing the physical exercises in this chapter, you have also proved to yourself the power of your thoughts on your body. This will give you the incentive you may need to take control of your thoughts rather than letting them control you.

Congratulations on taking your first step on the road to becoming younger.

> 'What a marvellous thing is youth. What a pity it is wasted on the young'
>
> George Bernard Shaw (1856–1950)

Change Your Beliefs

'Man is what he believes'

Anton Chekhov (1860–1904)

Before we begin, I need to be sure you have completed the written exercises for Step One in your notebook. If not, please go back and complete them now. You should only move on to Step Two once you have fully completed Step One, as this is a process that is designed to change your thinking and ageing step by step. You must complete each step systematically before moving on to the next one.

In this chapter you are going to learn that:

- You won't believe it when you see it.
- You will see it when you believe it.
- What we see and believe we become.

In Step One we worked on your thinking, now in Step Two it is time to work on your beliefs. 'Aren't thoughts and beliefs the same thing?' I hear you saying. Well, no they are not quite the same thing. Many people think one thing and believe another, so their mind is in a form of conflict. It is very important that your thoughts and beliefs are congruent, that they match and work together so that they complement each other, especially if you want to grow younger.

Our thoughts and beliefs are in conflict

Your thoughts and beliefs can be different and might therefore conflict with each other. If, for example, you think that you want to be wealthy although you believe that rich people don't ever know who their friends are or that money brings problems, or if you would love to get married although you believe that marriages don't last, or that men and women are always unfaithful in the end, these are all conflicting thoughts and beliefs.

A thought is something we hold in our minds, that we shape and form in our brain using language and pictures. Beliefs, on the other hand, can be so silent, and yet immediate, that we are not always aware that they are even there, yet they are absolutely influencing us; for example, if you believe that you are scared of dogs, your body will react to that belief as soon as you see a dog without you having to think about it at all. Your belief will set off an immediate reaction of fear within your body. It may react by having palpitations, shaking, sweating and even feeling sick. At the same time your thoughts may be busy saying, 'It's only a little dog. It's on a lead, it can't harm me, it's far away.' But your thoughts alone are having little or no impact on your belief.

It is the same with our beliefs about ageing. We may not be aware of them, they are somewhat silent, but we react to them very strongly, and they influence us 24 hours a day, which is why you will be doing an exercise on uncovering beliefs. It may seem somewhat similar to the exercise you did in the previous chapter, but in fact it is quite different.

Question, and doubt, your beliefs

We can change our thoughts quite easily with practice and repetition, but beliefs can take a little longer. The way to change a belief is to introduce doubt. If you have any beliefs you want to change, start to question where they originate from and ask yourself why you are holding them. Begin to introduce doubt to their validity. As soon as you question a belief, you are voicing doubt and you will no longer fully hold that belief to be true. The more you question a belief the more you will doubt it.

This book will enable you to doubt and question much that you have been taught about ageing. As you doubt your old beliefs, your mind will be receptive and open to accept new beliefs that will have a much more beneficial effect on your ability to age differently and to stay young. It can sometimes take only seconds for a belief to change, which is one of the reasons films with a twist in the tale are so popular – we believe one thing throughout, but at the end our beliefs are challenged and changed.

So, just to recap, to change your beliefs you must question where they came from and why you believe them now, or why you ever believed them at all. This questioning will make you start to doubt your beliefs. As soon as you challenge a belief you are ready to replace it because you no longer fully believe it. The more you challenge a belief, the more you are ready to replace it. This programme will show you how to doubt and challenge so many things that you previously accepted as truths about ageing. You will let go of old outdated beliefs as your mind accepts, in their place, new beliefs based on new facts, that will influence your ability to remain younger throughout your life.

BELIEFS ARE CHANGING ALL THE TIME

It can sometimes only take seconds for a belief to change. Look at the example of historic runner, Roger Bannister. It had been accepted and believed since records began that a human could not run a mile in under four minutes. Bannister was determined to change this, and he began by changing his own belief system. First, he saw the four minutes as 240 seconds, and then repeatedly visualised himself running a mile in 239 seconds. He used a form of self-hypnosis and visualisation to do this, and changed the general belief system about the mile. Within one year, 37 more people ran a mile in under four minutes, followed by 300 runners the following year.

There are examples all around us of people who have held a belief to be true for years, and then overnight their belief system changed. People might discover that a partner has been unfaithful or that their father is not their biological parent. More positively, people who have been told that they can't have children become pregnant, and people who don't believe in God change their belief immediately and permanently when something miraculous happens. We used to believe the earth was flat; we have since learned that this is not true.

Until recently we believed that Lance Armstrong was a uniquely gifted athlete, but the doping scandal changed that belief universally. The 2012 London Paralympics changed our beliefs about what disabled people could do and how they are viewed. It was wonderful to see athletes like Johnny Peacock receiving sex-symbol status despite losing their legs. Ellie Simmonds and David Weir were hero-worshipped along with many other amazing and inspiring athletes. In contrast, Jimmy Saville was once seen as a hero but is now loathed and despised.

As with thoughts, our beliefs are ours to change. Even definite and rigid beliefs can be changed. In the area of ageing you have nothing to lose, and everything to gain, by deciding to continually assess and review your beliefs, and from now on to hold beliefs about ageing that will be beneficial to you and which will empower you rather than disempower you.

BE FLEXIBLE ABOUT BELIEFS AND LEARN FROM OTHER CULTURES

There are different types and intensities of belief. There are beliefs that are opinions and beliefs that are convictions. Someone who is deeply religious would have a conviction. This is not open to doubt or change, because it would be stronger than an opinion. The reason for this is that in religion we are taught not to doubt but to accept without question the teachings of whichever religion we hold. If you want to age really well, you must be flexible about what you choose to believe rather than being rigid and inflexible. We must challenge all negative beliefs about ageing, since they are not based on facts and are most definitely not based on any facts that would be relevant to us.

Many primitive tribes are completely free of the signs of ageing that are accepted as normal in the Western world. In certain areas of the world, including China, Japan, India, the Hunza area of Pakistan, Georgia in Eastern Europe, Ecuador and parts of South America, people routinely live to be 100-plus and are very active. They still work, swim and exercise and are very involved in life. They have a very different belief system about ageing and are respected, revered and valued

Ken Hom, the famous Chinese cook and author, says, 'In China they believe you are nothing until you are 70; they value an older person's experiences because they can learn so much from them.' Since old age is looked up to in these cultures, people believe that as you grow older you grow in wisdom and esteem, and consequently they look forward to getting older and see it as a welcome age, with many advantages and privileges. Because of these different beliefs they live longer, healthier lives and they look and feel much younger than their years.

In a Harvard study that looked at people in Russia who lived very long lives, the researchers were surprised to find that Russians envied old people and saw old age as glamorous, which, they concluded, had a very real effect on their longevity. If you grew up in Japan and saw people reaching the age of 100, practising t'ai chi on a street corner every morning and being actively involved in life, you would see that as normal and would probably expect to age in the same way – and you probably would. Any changes you make in how you age must be preceded by a belief or thought that it will work or can work. Famous people and film stars are great examples at proving to us that what we have been led to believe about ageing can be contradicted.

DO YOU NEED WEALTH TO BE YOUTHFUL?

Sometimes, when I am lecturing, people tell me that it isn't fair to use, say, Joan Collins as an example of still being alluring at 81, or Honor Blackman, who is fabulous at 89, because of all the advantages someone in their position has. I completely understand this, yet there are many women out there who look just as fabulous and are doing it without the financial advantages of being a celebrity. I meet them all the time; however, since they aren't famous, we can't use them as examples. But they exist and are increasing in numbers almost daily. You can join them by using the techniques in this book.

How we age can be changed

When I was in the midst of writing this book, a participant at one of my lectures asked me, 'How can we stop ageing? Isn't it inevitable to age?' And I said, 'Well, yes in a way it is. From the moment we are born we are ageing and getting older, but rather than dispute that we age, the point is to question *how* we age and even *why* we age and what we *believe* about ageing.' Some species, for example salmon, are programmed to age rapidly and then to die very shortly after they have spawned, so really they only live long enough to procreate, whereas parrots and eagles have been shown to live for up to 50 years longer if they are removed from the elements. Meanwhile, Galapagos tortoises can live for 200 years without any help. Humans are not programmed to age or die after procreation, since they can have children in their twenties and still be fit and active in their seventies and eighties.

Ageing may be inevitable, but the way we age is far from inevitable. After all, if you were to study a cross-section of women in their late sixties they would all be ageing quite differently and to their own timetable. If we included Goldie Hawn (68), Sally Field (67), Diana Ross (70) and Lauren Hutton (70) in that cross-section of people, we would have absolute proof that ageing as we think we know it is not inevitable. Before you say, 'Oh, but they are all an exception', again I would ask you, 'How do you know that they are not an example of normal ageing and it is everyone else that is an exception?' With every belief you have about ageing, it is important to ask yourself:

- Where did that belief come from?
- Where did I get that belief from and what authority did the person who held that belief have?
- Where did they get it from and is it relevant to me?
- Is it based on anything that is real and tangible?

You may surprise yourself with some of your answers.

ROLE MODELS PROVE WE CAN AGE WELL

Beliefs related to ageing are changing all the time. Thirty-five years ago it would have been unthinkable to have female sex symbols in their late thirties. Now it is accepted – and 30 is seen as really young. In fact in a recent poll of Hollywood's most desirable women, Sharon Stone, Michelle Pfeiffer, Madonna, Meryl Streep and Cher were in the top ten. Susan Sarandon looked wonderful collecting an Oscar aged 50, Felicity Kendall appeared naked on stage also aged 50, Cherie Lunghi looks gorgeous at the age of 60 and looked so youthful when she danced on *Strictly Come Dancing*. Marie Helvin modelled bikinis in the year that she became 60 and Christie Brinkley appeared in *Chicago* playing the lead part of the young femme fatale, Roxie Hart, at the age of 58. Catherine Deneuve and Lauren Hutton were both modelling for major cosmetic and fashion companies at the age of 69.

Society has accepted this as no longer unusual, and it doesn't need to be unusual. Diana Ross, Cherie Blair, Annie Leibovitz, Jane Seymour and Susan Sarandon all had babies in their mid forties. Sophia Loren posed for the cover of the Pirelli calendar at the age of 71, Helen Mirren is a sex symbol at 68, Linda Gray looks sensational and sexy at 73, Bruce Forsyth is 86 and still compères *Strictly*. Alan Sugar is 67, Sir Robert Winston is 73, and they are both on our televisions as well as being active businessmen. Jane Fonda has recently released another book and another workout regime at 76.

We can find an example to contradict every belief about ageing that exists. Barbara Cartland and Catherine Cookson continued to write books every year well into their nineties; they never allowed their age to stop them. The famous author Mary Wesley wrote her first best-selling novel at the age of 70 and went on to write eight more best-sellers. When at the age of 84, with another book just published, she was asked how she could write such steamy sexual dialogue, she replied, 'Because I refuse to conform to the stereotype of an old lady.' She is an example to us that we don't have to lose our mental or physical agility at any age. Mary Berry, at the age of 79, is another wonderful example of this.

GREAT MINDS

If you have a reason to go on creating and to stay involved and active in life, your brain won't wither, because the brain does not wither when it is given new things to work on, and our mind never ages. Whereas most of us may have feared losing our agility and youth, would you dread ageing if you knew you would age like Katharine Hepburn, Martha Graham, Martha Gellhorn, Eileen Fowler or Freya Stark, who was still a writer and explorer at the age of 96 and who, like many people who aged well, found something that gave her the impetus and will to stay young? She triggered something in herself that made her third stage of life full of meaning and passion. The Queen is another wonderful example of this.

Most statistics about ageing have been carried out on people who were hospitalised and had not aged well, but there are just as many examples of people who have aged excellently and even took up climbing or running marathons in their seventies. I'm not suggesting you need to do that, but we can use these people as great examples, as role models. Here are some more:

- Artists Michelangelo and Pablo Picasso did amazing work in their late eighties and nineties respectively.
- Titian did his best work in his eighties and nineties.
- Verdi composed *Ave Maria* at 85.
- Martha Graham, the brilliant ballerina, was still performing on stage at 75, and at 95 she was choreographing her one-hundred-and-eightieth work.
- Lucian Freud continued painting until his death at 88.
- The pianist Vladimir Horowitz played to a sold-out Carnegie Hall at 98.
- Arthur Rubenstein did the same at 90.
- The Rolling Stones are still performing as they enter their seventies.
- Rod Stewart is still recording at 69.
- Nicholas Parsons, at 88, has great mental agility on the BBC Radio 4 programme *Just A Minute*.
- Bruce Forsyth is very agile and mentally sharp at 86.
- The cartoonist Ronald Searle survived years in a Japanese POW camp during the Second World War, proving that neglect earlier in life doesn't stop you from ageing well.

- William Gladstone was Prime Minister at 85 – and chopped trees daily.
- Oliver Wendell Holmes sat in the US Supreme Court into his nineties and said that faith in something keeps us young in spirit.
- Hulda Crooks began climbing mountains as she turned 70, and 25 years later made history when she became the oldest woman to climb Mount Fuji, which she did in her nineties.
- Judi Dench was amazing in the Bond film *Skyfall* at age 77.
- The Queen and Prince Phillip, Leo Tolstoy, Ormond McGill, George Burns, Katharine Hepburn, Jane Fonda, Iggy Pop, Betty Boothroyd, Bette Davies, Mary Wesley, Michael Heseltine, Lou Grade, Nicky Haslam and Mary Berry are all on the list of people who have retained their youth both physically and mentally.
- Fauja Singh took up running for the first time at the age of 80, and at the age of 100 has run several marathons.
- Daphne Self is the world's oldest model and works consistently at the age of 85.
- Baroness Trumpington, the Conservative peer, is still active in the House of Lords at the age of 91.
- Gillian Lynne, the ex-ballerina, still works full-time as a choreographer at the age of 87.
- Zhandra Rhodes is still designing fashion at the age of 73.
- Jilly Cooper recently published her latest book at the age of 77.
- Rosita Missoni retired and found she was bored, so she returned to work, founding and directing Missoni Home at the age of 82.

George Bernard Shaw said, 'Youth is wasted on the young.' You must believe that youth is a state of mind, that your body doesn't really age and neither does your mind, and that you have the power to choose to stay young throughout your life and to look and feel young too. Learn to welcome all the gains of maturity while remaining young, because you won't have lost anything unless you choose to believe that you have.

If you lose the natural desire for discovery and adventure – the childlike drive to do new things, to build and create and grow – if you just drift along, you will experience ageing at any age. We can, and must, keep finding attractive and exciting goals for the future. We may be tired of repetition, but it doesn't mean we are tired of life. You can be enthusiastic about life at any age, have goals that make you feel great about your future and about changing, have wide, varied interests and find things that allow you to feel excited about your future at any age – and you won't grow old. If you confront and change ideas that are not in harmony with youth, and instead become and stay active, alive and aware, you will remain young. You can only grow old if you stop growing: your brain and body won't shrivel when there are new things and new situations to keep them active.

Don't be taken in by media conditioning

Society and the media have preached, to women especially, a very limited view of ageing. The emphasis is often placed on worshipping youth and young bodies. Most of us would not even want to be back in our teens, because they are often full of angst and insecurity (teenagers have the highest suicide rate of all age groups), but we do want to look and feel young. We can choose to love the security that comes with maturity and believe that we look and feel better than ever – and make that our reality.

Recently, women have rebelled against this and have criticised the practice of having 17-year-olds modelling products aimed at 45-year-olds. In response to this, L'Oreal used Jane Fonda, at the age of 75, to model face cream. On a television show that was based around my book *Forever Young*, the host said that only rich people could remain young, that it had always been the case and that people without financial advantage could not slow down ageing. This is a belief, but if it were true then what about Nelson Mandela who spent 30 years in jail? He hardly had a privileged or wealthy life and yet his mental sharpness kept him youthful right up until his death.

It is so important not to believe negative conditioning about ageing. I am sure that being wealthy helps, but changing your thinking and your beliefs is free. Anyone can do it, and almost all the methods in this programme are either free or inexpensive.

Create good identify beliefs

Beliefs affect everything. Our identity beliefs – which are beliefs that we hold to be true about ourselves – affect what we do, where we go, how we dress, how we live and our choice of friends and careers. These are the most important beliefs. They can be empowering or limiting, depending on how we formulate them, since the strongest force in humans is the need to remain consistent with how we define ourselves.

Never define yourself by how old you are in years or allow anyone else to. Always define yourself positively. Look at the ways you define yourself, notice the language you use when describing yourself and change any definitions that aren't positive. If you do this enough it becomes a way of life; for example, be more like Sara, below, than Jill:

- **Jill** would believe, 'I look awful first thing in the morning', but **Sara** would change that to, 'I wake up looking rested and refreshed and good.'
- **Jill** would say, 'I look dreadful without make-up', but **Sara** would change that to, 'Make-up makes me look even better.'

Beliefs actually create biology. There is nothing in the world more powerful than our thoughts. No drug exists that is stronger than the mind. Beliefs are physical and real. Unfortunately, most people are completely unaware of the power of the mind. Unless you take charge of your thoughts and beliefs, you will be acting and reacting to the beliefs fed to you by others, which may have no relevance to you.

I want you to use the power of your mind to stay young. I am going to spend some of this chapter proving to you just how powerful your mind is, so that you can use it to slow down ageing, before I move on to show you how to use your mind consistently to look, feel and become younger.

By completing this very simple exercise, you will be able to experience how your beliefs cause physical changes to occur within your body.

Exercise 4: You can influence your body with your belief system

1   Stand up. Hold one arm with your finger pointing out in front of you, and begin to swing your arm as far out and behind you as you can. If it's your right arm, swing it out to the right and then as far behind you as you can; if it's your left arm, swing it out to the left and then as far behind you as you can. When you have moved your arm as far behind you as you can, look behind you to notice where it is.

2   Now, return to the starting position. Close your eyes for a moment, and just imagine your arm moving 25 per cent further. See this extra flexibility clearly in your mind for a moment, and tell yourself that when you repeat the exercise your arm will move 25 per cent further behind you. Then open your eyes, repeat the procedure, and notice just how much further your arm will move.   ▶

3   You are already beginning to see the power of beliefs on the body. As you saw, believed and thought about your arm moving further, it did. Repeat the exercise with the other arm to prove to yourself how easy it is to influence your body using your belief system.

Athletes have been using this technique of seeing themselves for years, to be able to lift a heavier weight or perform a longer jump, for example. By believing they can do it and will do, they are then able to do exactly that. Many tests have proven that in athletics, the ability to visualise is as important as physical training. When athletes visualise, they cause all their muscles to perform at a level to meet the visualisation. It is now becoming accepted that athletes who use powers of visualisation, as well as training, will always achieve more.

I once made a television documentary with some of my clients who are Olympic athletes. They were talking about how many athletes at the last Olympic games used the power of thought, belief and visualisation to succeed, and how it gave them an advantage over those who didn't, often helping them break a world record.

You may have heard stories of people who are slightly built or unfit, who have lifted a heavy object such as a car, a tree or a refrigerator off their child who has been trapped underneath, and then wondered how they managed it. In fact, they momentarily saw themselves performing the feat and then performed it, because in their mind, in that moment, they believed they could, and would, do it. One of the rules of the mind is 'imagination is more powerful than logic'.

The role of imagination in being healthy

Reason can be overruled by imagination, and you can use this to your advantage as you believe in your ability to influence how you age – and then make it a reality. People who see themselves as being ill, who believe they are ill, can and do manifest all the symptoms of illness, whereas people who refuse to see themselves as ill, or who won't believe they are unwell, frequently defy medical opinions. People who are ill but see themselves recovering and who use their imagination to see their cells becoming healthy, tend to recover much more rapidly than those who use the same powers of imagination and belief to focus on what is wrong with them. The people who recover quickly dwell on wellness instead of illness.

A phantom pregnancy is an obvious example of thoughts and beliefs in the mind creating physical changes in the body. During a phantom pregnancy, breasts can produce milk, the stomach will swell and, should the phantom pregnancy continue to full term, labour can begin, although only blood is passed.

Adoptive mothers are able to lactate and breast feed an adopted baby by visualising milk flowing into their breasts, and by wearing formula milk in a pouch with a tube running to their nipple so that as the baby sucks the milk it sends a powerful message to the brain to make more for feeding the baby. One of my clients, who adopted a three-week-old baby, immediately felt such love for it that she noticed when she was taking a bath the following week that her breasts were producing milk (and she had not even been on the lactating programme).

Another fascinating example of the power of belief on the body is that of people with multiple personality disorders, where one personality may have allergies or need glasses or have arthritis while another personality within the same person is completely free of these needs and afflictions. Some female multiple personalities have even switched on and off their periods depending on which personality they are experiencing.

These studies show us that cells are intelligent and make choices about how to behave below the level of our awareness.

Every cell in your body has its own micro brain. Cells accept what we tell them; they accept it when you say 'I am remaining young' or 'I am slowing down ageing'. If you constantly tell yourself that you are young or youthful, you are more likely to delay ageing, because your body will believe you and will act accordingly.

Our beliefs change through time

As we have seen, your cells and your body respond to what you believe, but beliefs change all the time. Many people condition themselves by believing ideas that are outdated and inappropriate; for example, it used to be believed that having our teeth, appendix and tonsils removed as a matter of routine was beneficial. Now that belief has changed, and we have been made aware that it can be harmful to remove parts of the body for no reason. When false teeth first became available, they were a status symbol, and some young, wealthy people had all their teeth removed and replaced with false ones because of this belief. In the early 20th century, it was fashionable for young, wealthy brides to be given a full set of false teeth as a wedding present from their fathers-in-law.

My grandmother, who was a beauty, had all her teeth removed when she was 30, because she had migraines and her doctor believed this drastic action – a widely held and accepted medical belief at the time – would cure her. Many beliefs based on medical opinions change, because new discoveries and facts come to light. This is never more true than in the anti-ageing field.

Emile Coue was a French pharmacist who was in practice at the end of the 19th century and the beginning of the 20th. He noticed that when he was dispensing drugs, patients always did better when he gave them positive suggestions. Coue reasoned that each of us has two selves: a conscious self and an unconscious self. The conscious self, which you are aware of, has an unreliable memory, whereas the unconscious self has a marvellous memory. It registers, without our knowledge, the smallest events and the least important acts of our existence. Your subconscious is also credulous, and it accepts without reasoning what it is told, especially what you tell it, since it has no reason to doubt you.

Your unconscious is responsible for the functioning of all your organs. If your subconscious believes that you can influence how you age, it will react positively to this belief; however, if it has accepted a suggestion that ageing is inevitable and you can do nothing about it, you are more likely to age badly and prematurely. Any negative suggestions, which you may not be consciously aware of, will influence how you age. The only way round them is by positive conscious suggestions that are frequently repeated so that the mind receives them and begins to act on them. If your mind believes that you will age just like your parents did, you are more likely to do so. If your mother was Goldie Hawn or an active Japanese woman in her nineties, this is a good suggestion, but if your parents aged badly it's a bad suggestion. Our unconscious presides over all our actions, whatever they are. This is what we call imagination and, contrary to accepted opinion, imagination makes us act, even against our will. It is an absolute law of the mind that your imagination always beats your willpower. Imagination is far more powerful than knowledge, and emotion is more powerful than logic when dealing with our own minds and those of other people.

If I asked you to stand on a window ledge only inches from the ground, you could stand on it effortlessly because you would imagine it to be easy, and that you cannot fall to the ground, because the ground is only a step away. If, however, you imagine that window ledge is now high up on the outside of a skyscraper, you would be scared of standing on it in case you fell. You would become anxious and nervous and more likely to fall off. You could stand on that amount of space when it was near the ground because your imagination told you it was OK. Now your imagination is telling you that it is not OK but that you could fall and die, and the same imagination will stop you from doing it. Even if you were offered a lot of money to stand on a window ledge 50 storeys high, you would be unable to do so, because in your imagination you would see yourself falling, and in this scenario your will is powerless against your imagination. The fear is caused entirely by the picture that you made in your mind and the words that you are going to fall. This transforms itself instantly into fact, because your mind cannot tell the difference between fact and fiction, in spite of all the efforts of your will, the harder that you try not to fall, the more likely it is that you will fall. Your mind cannot hold two pictures at once, so in order for you to think of not falling, you have to see yourself falling.

Train your imagination

The aim of this book is to train your imagination, so that it sees you as younger and believes you will remain younger at every stage of your life. Your imagination is like an untamed horse – it is immensely powerful, and you have to go where it wants you to go. The problem is that your subconscious mind has been formed by suggestions given to you by other people, by the media, by things you have seen on television, read in magazines, or heard other people saying. You accepted the suggestions and are now acting on them without even knowing it. Now, by learning and understanding the healing powers of your mind, you will be able to take control of how you age and influence it so that you always look and feel younger than your years.

People who have very strong religious beliefs are good examples of the power of belief systems. There are people who have willingly chosen to die because of their religious beliefs and believe that doing so is an honour – this is an important part of Japanese and Islamic culture.

If you constantly tell yourself you are remaining young and that your cells are young, they will believe you and act accordingly – but, of course, the opposite is also true. I know you may be thinking that that can't work, but throughout this programme I will be giving you examples that prove that it does.

You may come across people who scoff at what you are doing and say, 'I don't believe it.' When they do, just smile to yourself and remember that your cells absolutely believe it, your cells believe you. Your body believes it and is already acting accordingly. That, really, is all that matters.

This programme is for *you* to become younger, but don't try to make anyone else move over to your new point of view unless they want to. Other people may want to hold on to their old beliefs, and this is their choice. The best way to influence people to change is to change yourself so that they see the difference in you and want to follow.

UNTRUE BELIEFS – WRINKLES AND AGEING SKIN

As we have seen, your cells and your body respond to what you believe, and beliefs change all the time, yet many people condition themselves by believing things that are outdated and inappropriate. The belief that our bodies wear out in our sixties or seventies is not true, nor is the belief that as we age everything goes into a decline, so think of some examples you know that show how beliefs change and how your beliefs have changed, and know that as you change your beliefs about ageing you can literally change how you age.

Even the belief that our skin begins to wrinkle and show signs of age from 30 years onwards is not true. Wrinkles don't actually need to appear before we are 60, and although genes and gravity are linked to their arrival, exposure to the sun is the real cause of them arriving prematurely. Only 10 per cent of ageing is natural or genetic. Ninety per cent of wrinkles are caused by the sun. Wrinkles at 30 and 40 years of age are a sign of sun damage, which accounts for 80–90 per cent of ageing and wrinkling, followed by the effects of smoking and pollution.

I had a client aged 50 from Iran who had spent most of her life covered from head to foot in the chador. Until she left Iran and came to England her skin had hardly ever been exposed to the sun. She had no wrinkles and the skin of a 25-year-old. I am not suggesting we need to cover ourselves from head to toe to stay young but that we can discount the belief that ageing is inevitable.

Using a good sun block 365 days a year will also dramatically slow down the rate at which your skin ages. If you want to maintain young skin, always use a sunscreen with UVA and UVB radiation protective filters, every day of the year, especially on the face, hands, neck and the chest and breastbone, which has the thinnest skin on the body. It works better if applied to damp skin.

Use a sun block with a sun protection factor (SPF) of at least 15 or higher. Moisturisers and foundations or bronzers that contain their own SPF will not have a high enough factor, so use a sunscreen underneath. If you always protect your skin from the sun, do make sure you take enough vitamin D in your diet or by taking a good supplement, as we absorb vitamin D from the sun and need at least 20 minutes' exposure on our face and arms in order to absorb it. One of the best things to do to protect your skin while absorbing vitamin D is to leave sunscreen off your upper arms so they can absorb the 20 minutes of sun needed.

If you want more proof of sun damage to exposed skin, compare the back of the wrist of your left arm with the skin on your inner right arm. Take your wrist and place it across your other arm at the inner arm near your armpit, compare the skin of the two different parts of the arms and notice how different the skin looks and how different it feels. The skin on your inner arm looks and feels younger than the skin on your wrist.

Pinch the skin on your inner arm between your thumb and forefinger, hold it for five seconds and then let it go. Now count the number of seconds it takes for the skin to return to its previous condition. Do the same thing to the skin on your hand and you will see a big difference in the time it takes and how the skin pleats. If this were because of ageing, our skin would look the same all over our body. The skin on your inner arm is how all your skin would look – and could look – if it had not been damaged, because this skin gets protected from the sun whereas your hands get the most exposure to the sun and can age ahead of us. Sunscreen can prevent ageing spots on the hands, but you must wear it daily and reapply every time you wash your hands. Try to use an organic brand wherever possible.

The next major contributor to ageing is smoking, which ages skin by at the very least 10 per cent. Between the ages of 30 and 40 a smoker's skin will age by 16 years. Smoking limits blood flow to the skin and reduces its ability to repair damage. It also causes an increase in damaging free radicals. Puckering the mouth to draw on a cigarette also creates deep mouth-to-nose lines and lines all around the mouth. Squinting and half-closing the eyes during inhaling causes premature crow's feet, because the skin is left with a memory when it is repeatedly pleated or folded, and this memory is a wrinkle.

WORK ON CHANGING YOUR BELIEFS

You can change your body by changing your beliefs; you can quite definitely and visibly slow down ageing by removing pre-conditioned beliefs of ageing. We may have expected and learned to age, but with all the new information available to us we can also expect and learn to slow ageing down, to age differently. I know some of you will find this fascinating whereas others may wonder why should that happen. How do I know that this is true – that I can slow ageing? Well, consider this. Bees are able to completely reverse their age hormonally, when it is necessary for the hive. When there are not enough young bees to do the work that they are needed for, older bees will reverse their ageing and become younger and do the work that is designated for young bees. If the hive moves or separates into two hives, the younger bees can become hormonally older and do the work of older bees.

Planarians, a group of flat worms, can completely regenerate lost body parts. If a planarian worm is sliced in half or lengthwise, it will grow back into two healthy worms. The Turritopsis nutricula, a kind of 'immortal' jellyfish, can actually turn off the ageing process so that when it reaches adulthood, it alters the structure of its cells and reverts to a juvenile, sexually immature form.

Now you know that even bees and jellyfish can slow down ageing, there really is no excuse for you not to do the same thing since you have so much more information available to you. Humans have the greatest awareness of ageing, and we can use this awareness to our advantage by deciding not to believe in the inevitability of ageing but instead to believe that we can positively influence how we age, not just now but throughout our lives.

Are you ready to move on to another exercise, because I want you to begin now to look at your ageing beliefs? It is very important that you stop and think about your beliefs and how they are related to how you are ageing. In fact, over the next few days and weeks, become aware of any self-limiting beliefs you hold regarding ageing, and remember: they exist only in your imagination, since we can always find examples to counteract these beliefs.

Begin to root out and eliminate these beliefs and replace them with more positive ones. The mind can only hold one thought at a time, so you can banish negative beliefs and replace them with positive ones, once you have identified them and realised you can choose what to believe or not. Just because something has held to be true for a relative, it does not have to be true for you.

Exercise 5: Transform others' negative beliefs

1   When you have a quiet moment, close your eyes and begin to recall your parents' and your grandparents' attitudes and beliefs about ageing. Keep your eyes closed and think deeply about this; allow yourself to uncover all the silent hidden beliefs that have been affecting you.

a   Did they focus a lot on being too old to do things anymore?

b   Did they retire and spend long periods of time in a chair or being inactive?

c   Did they dress or act older before they needed to, and was their language entirely directed towards getting older?

If they did, it's important for you to know that we all have 25,000 hours of conditioning fed to us by parents and other influential figures. To feel younger, you must begin to change your dialogue and change the beliefs about ageing fed to you by others, which you may still be playing back to yourself, seemingly unaware. Without even knowing it, you are playing back old tapes of beliefs that are not yours but someone else's, but they are affecting how you age right now. You need to replace these outdated beliefs with new material that will help you instead of limiting you.

2   What about your friends' beliefs about ageing, do they match your own? Do you believe the same things? Do you go along with what they have said

▶

just because they said it? Close your eyes and just allow yourself to hear all the things you have heard from your family and your friends about ageing.

3   Using your notebook, write out the attitudes and beliefs about ageing held by people who could have influenced you but which you are now ready to see as outdated.

4   Underneath each attitude or belief, write out something new, positive and appropriate to you. Copy out this list of your new beliefs and keep it to hand – add it to your phone and computer, stick it onto your mirror and repeat these new beliefs to yourself daily. Here are some examples:

Example A: My mother always told me that getting older meant getting fatter and out of shape. CHANGE TO: I don't have my mother's body and I maintain a fit and healthy body at every stage of life.

Example B: My grandmother believed that everything ached with age and that exercise was bad for old people. CHANGE TO: Chinese people practise t'ai chi at all ages and exercise has never been bad for them – and nor is it for me. I find an exercise routine I enjoy and incorporate it into my life.

Example C: My father used to say 'mutton dressed as lamb' about our neighbour who always dressed young, so I feel uncomfortable about being ridiculed if I wear young fashions. CHANGE TO: Perhaps he envied her; she was happy with the way she looked. I am able to wear clothes that look good on me. I won't

▶

wear dull, safe clothes just because of someone else's negative thought process. Keeping up to date with fashions allows me to feel and look younger.

Example D: My grandparents believed that old people need lots of rest. I seem to remember them always sitting in the same armchair and being inactive. CHANGE TO: I have learned through this book that our bodies do not wear out with age, it is inactivity that accelerates ageing. I love my grandparents, but they were misinformed and wrong.

Example E: My employer believed that young employees were more productive and enthusiastic. CHANGE TO: Older employees are more reliable, experienced and dedicated.

5 Now decide how you are going to think about age in relation to yourself and write out these new beliefs on a new page and adopt them; accept them as your beliefs from now on.

Remember that you can succeed or fail in your ability to remain young depending on:

- What you choose to believe.
- What you choose to hold in your mind as true or not true.
- What you choose to see as relevant to you or irrelevant to you.

You may find as you go through Step Two's written exercises that they seem very similar to those of Step One. In Step One you are discovering and confronting your own thoughts about ageing, whereas in Step Two you are discovering and confronting the beliefs about ageing passed on to you by other people.

Some of these may be the same, or very similar, but even if you find yourself writing out some things that are the same as Step One, keep going, because it is important to release every negative thought and belief before you move on to Step Three. In this exercise you can analyse where these beliefs came from, how you got them and why you believe them.

Summary – Step Two

So let's recap everything you have learned in this step.

- You have learned that something you may have held to be true for years is just an outdated belief.
- You have learned that to change any belief you need to introduce doubt, because when you question and doubt a belief you will no longer hold it to be true.
- You have seen how examples of people who are living long, full and youthful lives are able to change the beliefs you hold about ageing.
- By letting go of old beliefs and replacing them with new ones, changes will already have begun to take place within your body.

Remember that before you can move on to Step Three you must have completed all the exercises in Step Two. If you haven't already completed them, go back and do them now before you move on to the next step.

'Man's mind, stretched by a new idea, never goes back to its original dimensions'

Oliver Wendell Holmes (1809–94)

Change Your Language

'Words form the thread on which we string our experiences'

Aldous Huxley (1894–1963)

We are going to look at the power of language and its effect on ageing. Language and the words you use associated with ageing have a very powerful effect on the body and mind, because words have an emotional content and what we associate with the words we use shapes how we feel about things. Experiments have shown that if we take on someone else's emotional vocabulary we also take on their emotional state.

Years ago, while I was driving around London, I noticed the billboards advertising George Michael's new album; the title of this album was *Older* and it had a picture of George. I frequently heard the song on the radio, and the chorus says, 'Baby don't you think I'm getting older now?' It's not a sad song, it's very positive, because it's all about growing up and becoming mature, becoming a grown-up. But imagine if the song had been called 'Old' instead of 'Older' and the lyrics had been, 'Baby don't you think I'm getting old now?' with the billboards showing George Michael's picture and the word 'Old'. The word is only slightly different and yet the meaning and the connotation of the two words are so different. Old is generally seen as negative; older means wiser and smarter.

Words are very powerful, and the meaning we attach to them has a big influence on us.

People who have not aged well tend to complain and draw attention to their age or their aches and pains all the time and use words that are negative, whereas those who have aged well tend to draw attention to how well they feel and use much more positive language. To age well you must eliminate words like 'exhausted', 'worn out', 'shattered', 'depressed', 'sick', 'doddery' and 'past it', because the label or word you use to describe how you feel *becomes* how you feel.

Choose descriptive words with care

Our mind responds to and loves words that are descriptive, because it makes its work easier to do. So now that you know this, use only descriptive words that are positive. Words are the structure of our reality, and it follows that if we change our words we then change our reality. Certainly, making changes in the language we use changes very quickly how we feel. That's why it is vital to pay attention to our thoughts and language connected to ageing.

Our cells listen to, and react to, our language, so if you were to say, 'I'm too old to go to fitness classes any more; it's too exhausting for me', immediately your mind and body will accept this as factual, and thus, by believing you are too old, it will cause you to feel and act older than is necessary.

Making a very simple change to your language, however, will have a different effect on your body, such as saying, 'I'm too tired to go to fitness class today, so I will take it easy and go tomorrow.' Instead of saying 'I look old', decide to say, 'I look a little stressed or tired.' Instead of saying 'I am exhausted/worn out', choose to say, 'I need to enjoy some deep sleep so that I can look refreshed and relaxed.'

If you use ageing language, and if your identity of yourself is old or ageing, your DNA will pass on through each cell generation the belief that you are old or ageing. If your language and thoughts are all along the lines of 'I can't remember things like I used to' or 'I don't have the energy to do the things I used to do', you are passing on that information from one cell to the next. Cells are not able to disagree with you and they accept everything you say, or even think, as a fact, so you have nothing to lose and everything to gain by telling yourself and your cells the opposite. Tell yourself you look and feel ageless.

THE NEGATIVE ASSOCIATIONS WITH 'OLD' START EARLY

I noticed that even small children see the word 'old' negatively. When my daughter was five she was given an antique doll's house by her godparents, and when I showed it to people I would say, 'It's very old' or 'It's a hundred years old.' My daughter was really far too young to have been given it and would either try to get inside it or swing on the doors as they opened out. I must have said to her, 'Don't do that because this doll's house is very old' too many times, because one day she said to me, 'Mummy, why don't we get rid of that doll's house, it is so old, and get a pink Barbie house instead?'

That got me thinking about where she could have picked up the belief that old equals undesirable, and I noticed my language as I said things like, 'Throw away that fruit in the fridge – it's really old', or clearing out her room I would say, 'Do you want to keep all these old things? Or could we get rid of some of them?' And, of course, she heard me talk to other people and say to my husband, 'Don't wear that, it looks so old' or 'I need some new running shoes, these are really old now', or 'This DVD player is so old, we'll have to replace it.'

People value newness so much – children, especially, love having new things. Yet some of my favourite things are my oldest things, and my daughter certainly loved her oldest teddy bear the best. Since then, I endeavour not to equate undesirable things with their age. I now say, 'Don't eat that. It isn't fresh/it's gone off/it's mouldy' rather than saying it is old.

If you think about the context in which you use the word 'old' it may give you some insight into why so many people dread ageing. We value special objects that are old, yet we also use the word 'old' as a prefix for replacing something or discarding something, chucking it out, believing it no longer has any value.

The feeling of loss

In the area of language, the mind reacts very badly to the word 'loss', so if you mourn your lost youth and believe that your schooldays were the best days of your life, if you use expressions like 'It's all downhill from now on' or 'I am losing my looks', you will accelerate the ageing process.

The greatest human pain is all to do with what we believe we have lost. When people talk about losing their looks, or their hair or hair colour, or their agility, it feels so negative, but it doesn't have to. You need to see it as a *change* instead of a *loss*. Your looks are changing, but change isn't a bad thing – it can be a great thing. The only way you can stay the same is to have an illness that means you remain a child, and you wouldn't choose that. So although you are not going to stay exactly the same, you can focus on all the things that are positive about the changes in your life. The only thing you need to lose is the old beliefs that have been so detrimental to you. Now you can put your focus on maintaining a youthful attitude and approach to life at any age while gaining more knowledge, ability and desire to look after your body and your health.

Recognise the power of your thoughts

Work through the following quick exercise to see just how powerful your thoughts and words are.

Exercise 6: A fresh lemon

1   Imagine that you are standing in your kitchen and you are holding a lemon that you have just taken from the fridge. It feels cold in your hand.

2   Look at the outside of it: the yellow waxy skin that comes to a small green point at both ends. Squeeze it a little and feel its firmness and its weight. Now imagine raising the lemon to your nose and smelling that unique fresh lemon smell.

3   Now imagine cutting the lemon in half and inhaling it – the smell is stronger. Now imagine biting deeply into the lemon and letting the juice swirl around in your mouth. Taste the sharpness, the fresh citrus flavour. At this point, if you have used your imagination well, your mouth will be watering.

Consider the implications of this. Words, mere words, affected your salivary glands. The words did not even reflect reality, but something you imagined. When you read those words about the lemon you were telling your brain you had a lemon. Although you did not mean it, your brain took it seriously and said to your salivary glands, 'He/she is biting a lemon. Hurry, wash it away.' Your glands obeyed. If something as simple as imagining you were eating a lemon can cause your body to react physically, then something as simple as imagining you are slowing down the ageing of your body can, and will, cause your body to react physically.

Words do not just reflect reality; they can *create* it – like the flow of saliva you just caused by doing the exercise. The subconscious mind is no subtle interpreter of your intentions; it receives information and it stores it, it believes without question everything you tell it, since its job is not to question but to act immediately on your instructions, which to your subconscious mind are commands. Tell your subconscious mind something like 'I am eating a lemon' and it goes to work. That experiment was neutral, so physically no good or harm can come from it, but good as well as harm can come from many of the words we use.

Exercise 7: 'I am old and weak' vs 'I am young and vibrant'

Let's do some more exercises that will show you the power words have on your body. You will need someone to help you to do them.

1   Hold one arm out in front of you and clench your fist, making that arm as rigid and as strong as you can. Now get your helper to push down on that arm to test your strength while you use all your strength to resist them. As they try to push your arm down, resist them as much as you can.

2   Now you have established your strength, think of the most negative words you use about yourself in relation to ageing. Repeat these words out loud ten times or just think them silently ten times. An example could be 'I am old and weak' or 'I am constantly getting older and less desirable'.

▶

3   While thinking those words, make your arm rigid again and repeat the strength-testing process with your helper. Amazing isn't it? When you think those negative words you are losing all the strength in your muscles and your arm is becoming weak; you are weaker while thinking or saying those words.

4   To prove further that thoughts and words are even more powerful than effort in tests of strength, and to see for yourself the powers of your language on your body, this time think of some positive thoughts about ageing yet remaining young; repeat them out loud or silently ten times. If, like many of us, you have been led to believe that there is nothing positive about ageing, then repeat this ten times:

'I am remaining young, healthy and vibrant.
My body and mind are always young.'

5   Now, thinking these words, make your arm rigid again and repeat the strength-testing process. Isn't it great to see that as you think positive thoughts you become physically stronger? I mentioned earlier that every thought you have creates a physical reaction in the body, and you have just proved it to yourself.

Where a thought goes, energy goes with it, so you can see that changing your thinking and using different language really does change your body. Most people are fascinated by this test, and since it's a fun thing to do I recommend you spend some time playing with it by:

1 Repeating all the negative thoughts and beliefs you have. Using all the negative words you had been using before realising the power of language.
2 Testing your strength.
3 Replacing these beliefs with positive, constructive beliefs.
4 Testing your strength again and seeing the difference.

You can do this with so many beliefs, not only in the area of ageing but in beliefs you have about your confidence, self-esteem, your abilities, your relationships – in fact anything at all. Remember that these beliefs exist only in your imagination. You are free to change your thinking and your language as soon as you become aware of how limiting and destructive your language and beliefs are. Your thoughts are yours to change, your mind is yours to direct, and your language is yours to alter.

Fast results through changes in language

Although the mind does run the body, it is *your* mind and you are able to direct it, to change it, and to influence positive changes in yourself. Changing your language is one of the quickest ways to do this. Now we are ready to move on to some written exercises so, using a notebook, let's begin by thinking of all the words and language you use to describe yourself.

Exercise 8: Change negatives into positives

1 Write out all the words and language in your notebook that you use to describe yourself. Here's an example: you may frequently use words like 'old', 'too old', 'ancient', 'antique', 'over the hill', 'past it', 'gaga', ▶

'wrinkly', 'exhausted', 'worn out'. Keep on writing the words until you have found all the words you use.

2   Close your eyes and remember conversations you have and the words you use the most. Ask your friends, family and children what negative words you use most frequently.

3   When your list is complete, go through it and delete all the words that are not positive. Now find new words that are not negative and not so descriptive in a negative way to replace the ones you have deleted. Or you can just erase those words from your vocabulary without needing to replace them.

Never say, 'God, I look ancient' or 'I feel ancient', even in jest. Don't use words like 'geriatric', 'antique', 'past it', 'over the hill' or 'decrepit', because the way you are describing yourself is the way you are becoming. You can retain a youthful skin and fast and quick thinking through the power of your mind, but you won't if you keep using awful phrases like 'no spring chicken', 'old boiler' or 'old fogey' to describe yourself, even if it's only jokingly. Remember that your subconscious mind has no sense of humour and it takes everything you say literally. It's vital to laugh and to have a sense of humour, and it's OK to make fun of yourself, but not in the area of your age. Most people only joke about ageing because they feel uncomfortable about it.

Widen your vocabulary for the good things in life

There are over 750,000 words in the English language and most people only use 1,200 of them. Most people have the same 12 words that they use to describe their experiences and feelings. It is especially interesting to me that many people use very descriptive and powerful words to describe events that are mediocre but use words that are not powerful enough to describe good things that are happening to them.

Sometimes a patient will arrive at my office and say, 'I've had a hellish morning on the road', or 'The parking around here is a nightmare', or 'I've been stuck in the supermarket – it's torture in there', or even 'I've had the most appalling time getting here.' Then, just for good measure, they will add, 'My back is killing me' or 'I have starved myself all week, but I still look as fat as a house.'

Without realising it, they are using very powerful, descriptive words to describe events that aren't really that important and need to be forgotten, not elevated and remembered in the mind as scenes of hell, chaos, torture or a nightmare. Describing pain as 'killing' or 'crippling' can only intensify it. Saying you are 'ravenous' or 'starved' can cause you to over-eat because your mind will believe you *are* starved and will shut down your appestat, which controls how much you eat and tells you when you have had enough.

Saying 'My memory is like a sieve', 'I'm as deaf as a post', '. . . as old as the hills' or 'I'm geriatric' gives the mind a very clear image to move you towards.

When these same clients begin to talk about good events in their life or how they are feeling, they use words that are weak or not very descriptive, such as 'It was quite good', 'It was OK really', 'I had a nice time', 'It was fun', 'We had a laugh', 'It turned out all right', 'I'm not too bad', 'I'm OK', 'I'm all right', 'I'm fine.' These words are so un-descriptive, so vague and wishy-washy, that they fail to have impact on the mind. If you want to feel better, use words that are very descriptive and which make a picture that is thrilling or exciting and powerful.

Even the words you place in front of other words will have an effect on how you feel. This is especially true with swear words, which are used to intensify a feeling. If you say an event was awful but add in front of it that it was 'absolutely awful', 'bloody awful', 'fricking awful' or 'absolutely bloody, fricking awful', you get a stronger response in your mind and body to how awful it was and to how awful you feel it was. That is why we put the F-word in front of other words, because it intensifies the feeling and the description we are making.

If you say it was 'amazing' or 'fantastic', but then add '*truly* amazing', '*simply* amazing' or '*absolutely* amazing', you'll get a stronger reaction to the event, but this reaction is positive whereas the previous one was negative. If you describe yourself as a 'pig', then put in front of it 'I'm a big fat pig', your mind creates a much more vivid picture and a more intensified feeling accompanies those words. If you call yourself a 'doddery old fool' or 'as blind as a bat', your mind creates a vivid picture for you to turn into.

Exercise 9: Emphasise the positive

1   Think of the words you use the most frequently, both positive and negative, to describe yourself.

2   Write the positive words down the left-hand side of your notebook and the negative words down the right-hand side.

3   Now write them out again, but this time really increase the list of positive words and decrease the list of negative words. An example of this would be for you to write down:

'I am not bad looking.' This is not positive enough. Change it and accentuate it to, '*I look wonderful*.'
'I have frown lines.' This is negative, so minimise it to, '*They are character lines and tiny*.'

▶

'I am not bad for my age.' This is not positive enough, so change it and accentuate it to, '*I am an excellent example of ageless ageing.*'

'I get tired more often.' This is negative, so minimise it to, '*I rest more and then have abundant energy.*'

4   Now think of the words you use in front of words and decide to put words like 'absolutely', 'definitely', 'positively', 'unquestionably', and so on, in front of your new positive statement while using words of a different intensity, like 'slightly', 'mildly', 'occasionally', and so on, in front of negative statements.

Look afresh at the way you use negative statements

Don't use words with a strong negative emotional content. Never say things like, 'I am dreading being 50' or 'I can't bear to think of being a pensioner' or 'I loathe the thought of old age'. The more descriptive and negative those words are the more they will elevate in a negative way how you feel about ageing when it could become a wonderful time of life.

If you are used to saying 'I have horrible wrinkles all over my body', change it to 'I have a very slight amount of wrinkling in certain parts of my body, and no-one else really notices them'.

What your mind sees it believes without question. It has no capacity to reason. It therefore believes whatever you tell it, so you absolutely must get into the habit of telling yourself only positive things. Although your mind may doubt and question the things that others tell you, it will not doubt or question what *you* tell it, so become ultra-aware of the language and the words you use to describe things, most especially the words you use to describe yourself, because your mind particularly responds to words and images that are symbolic – the subconscious mind loves descriptive words. You are going to be like the thought police watching out for unacceptable words and removing them.

When you say 'I am knackered' or 'I am worn out' or 'I am a dinosaur in my office', your body works to meet the mind's description. Simply changing that to 'I am a little tired today' or 'I feel fatigued at the moment' or 'I have the most experience within my company' brings about completely different sensations. Calling wrinkles 'laughter lines' and 'character lines' does this. Do not call them 'crow's feet' – that is such a hideous description. When Leslie Caron was having her picture taken, she said, 'Please don't airbrush out my lines. I have worked so hard to earn them.' She attached pleasure rather than pain to them and was quite proud of them.

When I hypnotise clients to give birth I remove the words 'labour', 'pain' and 'contractions' from the conditioning CD I make for them and instead talk about 'delivery', 'birth signals', 'rushes', 'feelings', 'sensations', 'euphoria'. Many of my clients who listen to this CD during the last stages of pregnancy and during delivery say they love it because it contains no negative words and allows them to experience childbirth in a more manageable way. When I was pregnant I was amazed that my antenatal clinic wanted to remind me at every visit to be prepared for post-natal depression, and I would always reply that I was going to have post-natal euphoria. I didn't mind them talking about it, and I understood the need to be informed about this, but they talked about it so much, with such fervour, that eventually I stopped going. They always seemed to go into so much detail about the pain of birth, the baby blues and the exhaustion of being a new mother. Because I am so aware of the power of language, I was not prepared to hear and absorb so many negative words on such a regular basis.

I had a very easy pregnancy and birth, and I did have post-natal euphoria. I was on a high after my baby was born and I had so much energy and felt fantastic and so happy. Some of this was natural, and a lot of it was to do with the fact that I had conditioned myself to believe different things. I used different language and thought different thoughts. I also had great motivation to do this, since I knew that three weeks after my baby's birth I would be on live television demonstrating hypnosis for childbirth with a lady who was phobic about hospitals, and I took my baby on the programme with me. I was regarded as somewhat of an exception, because I returned to my normal weight in a week and I felt fantastic. I still believe that a lot of the things we hear about pregnancy – the weight that takes a year to go, the tiredness, the depression – can also be negative conditioning that many women react to automatically because of the way the mind works. And it's the same with ageing. We hear so much that is bad about it and yet most older people would not choose to return to their youth, if given the opportunity; they would just like to go back by about ten years, and you can do that using the power of your mind.

Persistence is key

You may need to persist with changing your language and vocabulary if you have been using powerful and negative words to describe yourself or your feelings for some time. The mind learns by repetition and by a new process of positive repetitions. Using much better language, you will see and experience definite changes.

Using this programme, and these examples, will show you how to:

- Take control of how you age.
- Challenge ageing beliefs.
- Re-create your thoughts and beliefs regarding ageing.
- Change your attitudes, awareness and language connected to ageing.
- Commit to feeling young and living a young life.

When you have finished this book you will be able to take control of how you age, as opposed to being helpless and letting ageing just happen to you. You will be able to take charge of ageing rather than giving up and expecting a decline into ageing. Most of us only really fear and resist change in case we become worse off. We fear ageing because we are taught that everything about it is bad, there is nothing good, so we see it as a loss and hugely negative, but it does not have to be that way. You don't have to dread ageing, because changing years is not ageing. This book will help you to take control of the direction of ageing and to assure you that the direction of all change is towards improvement so that you can feel good about yourself at every age. It's hard to feel good about ourselves unless we feel that we are influencing the direction of change in our lives. When you are influencing the change and seeing that some of those changes are changes for the better, you can feel good about yourself.

Don't wish, hope or dream of ageing well. Instead, *know* that you will make that a reality for yourself. *Believe* that you will make that happen for you now. *Know* that it will happen.

When you wish for something you send a message to the brain that says, 'I want this, but I don't believe I can ever have it.' When you say, 'I will try', your brain immediately accepts the word 'try' as so insignificant that it does not matter if you get the results or not. When you say, 'I will' instead, you get a very different and positive response. Saying 'I hope it works' allows your mind to believe that you doubt that it will work. Saying 'I can only dream about staying young' is interpreted by the mind as dreaming about something because you have already accepted it is not attainable or going to happen.

OUR MINDS PREPARE OUR BODIES FOR HEALING

Some years ago I was asked to work with a little boy who had eczema. His parents were very keen that he might find a cure for this before he started school, whereas his grandmother, who lived with the family, would comment frequently that they should all stop fussing, since it would go away anyway once he started school. I could not give them an appointment until after he had begun his first term at school, as I was working abroad. Interestingly, as soon as he began school the eczema started to diminish, and by the time he arrived for his appointment it was already improved by 75 per cent, because he had accepted his grandmother's words and his mind had acted upon them. Occasionally, clients book appointments with me to help them stop smoking or biting their nails and when they arrive for the said appointment they have often already stopped or considerably reduced the habit, because they expected to, and in a sense they saw it happening.

I have my own personal experience of the power of thought. Having been told I couldn't have children, I went on to get pregnant very easily, helped by the fact that I did not ever accept the diagnosis that I would be childless. I would not allow myself to picture myself as childless, and as my doctor was trying to explain why I could not have a baby I remember saying to him, 'Don't tell me that.' I just refused to accept it, or even hear it. I knew I had to not let my mind take in what he was saying, and I'm so glad I didn't, because now I have a wonderful daughter. I used hypnosis throughout my pregnancy and had the easiest pregnancy, an easy birth and a baby who was content and hardly ever cried.

I was put on thyroid medication for years and was told that I could never come off it and could not get pregnant with or without it, but I became pregnant and decided after my daughter's birth not to take any more medication. With the help of a wonderful doctor, who believed I did not need the medication, I came off it easily and have never felt better. I should mention here, however, that if you are on any prescription medication, only come off it under the guidance of a doctor.

YOUR MIND CAN MAKE DOING DIFFICULT THINGS EASIER

Many years ago I went on a training course in Hawaii that involved walking on burning coals and climbing 15m (50ft) telegraph poles. Before I left England I decided that I would pass on the pole-climbing. I stood on the edge of the roof of a building that was 15m up and didn't like it very much. I noticed that I was saying to myself, 'I'm not going to climb the pole.' When I arrived in Maui and saw other people climbing the poles I declined and told the organisers that I didn't want to do it and I had no intention of doing it. And then on my last day but one, I watched a little girl of five climb the pole, and this immediately changed my thinking. I decided that if she could do it so could I. As I changed my thinking everything changed – I began to want to do the climb. I started to feel excited about it. A few hours later I was standing on top of the pole balancing on one leg having my photograph taken – it was wonderful and thrilling, I loved every moment of it, and it was a wonderful lesson to me on changing my thinking and changing my feelings. I will always be grateful to that little girl. After that, the fire walking was easy. At one time I would never have gone on a course like that, but I'm so glad I did, because it opened my eyes even more to the amazing power of the mind over the body.

Programmes like *I'm a Celebrity … Get Me Out Of Here* show us the same ability to make a mental shift, which then changes everything. When the celebrities decide it is in their interest to eat bugs or animals' genitals or to shower in worms and spiders, they can make themselves do previously unthinkable things sometimes with apparent ease. One of my clients was jailed in Africa and said that during the first few days the rice was so full of worms she could not eat it, but after a few weeks she became so desperate for protein that she ate the worms first and would have been disappointed if the rice came without them.

Summary – Step Three

Let's recap everything you have learned in Step Three.

- You have learned the power of language, the very real and physical effects your words have on your body.
- You have learned that some of the most simple and easy changes are the ones that will have the most lasting impact on the body.
- You have learned that the words you say to yourself have more impact on how you age than the words you hear others say.
- Changing your language is such an easy thing to do once you get started.

You are almost a third of the way through the programme and are well on the way to noticing changes beginning to occur in how you feel and how you look.

> 'As you speak you are and as you continue to speak so you remain'
>
> Anonymous

Find and Change Your Biological Age

'People don't grow old. When they stop growing they
become old'

Anonymous

In this step you are going to learn how to make your body feel
younger, because, as you know by now, this will actually lead
your body to becoming younger. Making your body feel younger,
and consequently become younger, is very easy to do, and you
need only spend a few minutes every day, or 10–15 minutes three
or four times a week, to get the desired results and to keep them.
Your muscles have a memory, which can be activated by your
beliefs and physiology. You never forget how to ride a bike, for
example, because it is in your physiology.

Change your habits and stay childlike

Doing things you did when younger not only reminds your muscles how to behave and what to do but they also remind your cells
that this is the activity of a youngster. As we participate in young
behaviour and young activities, our cells feel, act and ultimately

behave younger. Swimming, skipping and rebounding on a mini trampoline are excellent examples of activities that can slow down the age of our cells. Cycling also works, if you activate memories of being a child while cycling for fun; riding a stationary bike hard in the gym won't have the same effect.

It's important to exercise if you want your body to look and feel younger, but taking exercise to remain fit and supple and to have stronger bones is not what I am talking about here. Even if you regularly exercise by running, weight training or practising yoga, you still need to participate in other activities that are designed to make you feel young, because these will remind your body what it was like being a child rather than giving your body a workout.

There are some activities, like swimming, jumping and skipping, that do both, but when you engage in these in order to keep fit they usually take an hour or so and lose the aspect of spontaneous fun over extended periods of time. Although we might still enjoy them they can become competitive as well. To become biologically younger, separate exercising for the benefit of keeping fit from moving in a childlike way.

I go to the gym and practise yoga to keep supple and in shape, but I separate those from the times when I dance around or jump up and down to activate a feeling of being young. When you exercise regularly, it can cause you to become young biologically because of the physical effect exercise has on your body and on your muscles. When you regularly engage in young activities that are fun, this in turn will cause you to feel young, which is transmitted to your organs and can cause you to become physically younger, because it is influencing your psychological age.

Rebounding or trampolining regularly for 10–20 minutes three or four times a week is an important anti-ageing tool. It is excellent for cells and age reversal, because rebounding stimulates your production of lymph, which is essential for looking and feeling healthy. We have more lymph in our body than we have blood; however, the lymph does not have a pump, so we need to take regular deep, diaphragmatic breaths and move a lot to allow the lymph to move around the body. Muscle movement and gravity are meant to keep lymph flowing, pump lymph back through its channels and eliminate waste. Running, rebounding, jumping, skipping, swimming and other forms of aerobic exercise encourage correct lymph activity and flush wastes from tissue fluids. Using a rebounder, which is also known as a mini trampoline, for just a few minutes daily is excellent for promoting correct lymph movement.

We eliminate waste through our skin, lungs, kidneys and colon. Up to a third of waste elimination is through the skin. Our sweat glands are meant to expel a minimum of one pound of waste material daily. When they don't because our bodies are not working at peak efficiency this toxic waste can remain in our system causing all kinds of damage and accelerating ageing. James White, an exercise physiologist in California, put a group of previously inactive older women on a rebounding programme and noted that those on the rebounders looked younger than the control group that remained inactive. Their skin tone and colouring improved, their wrinkles diminished and so, to his amazement, did the bags under their eyes – and these changes occurred within a matter of weeks. Another benefit with rebounding is that while we are bouncing on a trampoline to some fun music, we feel like children, and when we are feeling young psychologically, this will make us younger biologically.

Youthful music

As you bounce, it is excellent to think positive thoughts, to repeat the affirmations that you will learn about in Step Five, and to listen to some music with anti-ageing lyrics, such as *Young at Heart* by The Bluebells. Sing some lyrics or affirmations out loud. Your new beliefs will go directly into your subconscious mind and influence you in the most perfect way. Jumping or skipping is excellent for boosting your lymphatic system, and swimming is perfect because the combined action of water and muscle movement stimulates the lymphatic system. It's as good as rebounding and better for people who have joint, weight or heart problems.

There are other ways of making your body first feel younger and then become younger, such as giggling or laughing out loud – even playing board or card games from your past can evoke the feelings of youth and then stimulate the desired effect of feeling, and ultimately becoming, younger.

Moving around to some music that you particularly like is equally excellent for making your body believe it is younger in order to physically become younger. Music from the past instantly regresses us to our past. If we hear the music that was played on our first date, at our first dance, or the music we fell in love to, it takes us back to that time. It's important to only play music that evokes happy memories that make you smile, laugh or sing, so don't play those sad break-up records, because they won't do you any good at all.

Find some songs that have the word 'young' in them and make a point of playing them daily; set aside a few minutes and dance to them every day. It will make you feel great. Have your favourite as your ring tone on your phone. Any fun music or rhythmic music that you love will do; however, if you listen to some of my recommended songs listed below, especially if you play them over and over, you will find the lyrics become embedded in your mind. Messages combined with music bypass the conscious and go straight into your subconscious. You will be able to use the appropriate lyrics as affirmations, hearing the positive messages they contain being played back to you again and again. You could even sing them out loud, and you will be taking another positive step to feeling and becoming younger. Here are some of my favourite anti-ageing songs that I play at my seminars:

Young at Heart by Frank Sinatra
Young at Heart by The Bluebells
You Make Me Feel So Young Frank Sinatra

Forever Young by Bob Dylan and also by Chrissie Hynde
Young Turks (Young Hearts Be Free Tonight) by Rod
  Stewart
Young Gifted and Black by Bob and Marcia
When You're Young and in Love by Tammi Terrell
Young Hearts Run Free by Candi Staton
Be Young, Be Foolish, Be Happy by The Tams
Alright (We are young, feel alright) by Supergrass

If you know of any other titles with the word or theme 'young' in them, please email me and let me know what they are, as I play these songs during the breaks at my seminars and love having more titles to use.

Falling in love

When we fall in love we become very childlike, because falling in love is an act of regression, so we act much more like children. We become spontaneous and carefree, we touch and explore, rub noses, talk in baby talk, hold hands, cuddle up, find pleasure in the most simple things and notice that time stands still and that we become absorbed and focused on one thing, oblivious to all else. These are all qualities that children have. We dance around and smile a lot – even at total strangers – we laugh more, we sing to ourselves and feel content. While we are doing this are bodies are literally growing younger, and falling in love also makes us look visibly better.

BE IN LOVE WITH LIFE – LIKE A CHILD

Although you may not be in a position to just fall in love, you could put yourself in a position of recreating the feelings and remembering how it felt to be in love, and then recreate some or all of those feelings. Children seem to be in love with life. They can find pleasure in the rain and wind, in a puddle or a rainbow; just seeing a snail or a spider's web delights them – they can make anything and everything an adventure. We can learn a lot by remembering that we once had all those qualities, and it is never too late to reclaim them. As we grow up we get wrinkles, but the worst place to have wrinkles is in your enthusiasm. It does not matter if your face has wrinkles as long as your enthusiasm is unblemished.

Children are naturally spontaneous, creative and flexible. One day when I was taking my daughter to school, I noticed a large puddle in the playground and most of the mothers were saying, 'Don't go in that puddle. Don't get your feet wet.' One little boy ran up with glee straight into the puddle where he happily splashed, soaking his shoes and socks while his mother looked on exasperated. When children come across puddles they jump in; when adults come across them they moan and complain about them. Sometimes we need to be childlike and jump in the puddle as well. When we do it feels so good, we get to understand again why children love to do this kind of thing and we get to feel more like them.

When I was walking down our street with my daughter, she said, 'Mummy I've never seen you run or skip along this road. Please skip with me.' Because it was important to her and I was in a carefree mood, I took her hand and, feeling a bit foolish, I skipped along the road with her.

I was doing this solely for her, but I noticed after a few minutes how good it felt. We were giggling and laughing and I felt so young and childlike. Of course, I knew what a great effect this was having on my cells and on my psychological and therefore my biological age, and I vowed to do it more often.

There are other times, of course, when I have no desire to do this. I don't want to be in the park or playing and I want to be serious and adult, left alone to read the papers. It's all to do with being appropriate. Do childlike things when you can, but don't wait for the mood to hit you – *make* it happen as well.

Every time it's been my daughter's birthday and I've hired a bouncy castle, the adults can't wait to have a go on it once the children are elsewhere. There is something about that party environment – the balloons, the children's food and giggling, the clown entertainer, the music and that carnival-like atmosphere – that makes us regress back to childhood for a few delightful moments. I believe we should be encouraged to do this more, not less, because of the positive effect it has on our cells. Sometimes when you go on the swings or the slide or the roundabout in the park or you splash in the paddling pool with your children or grandchildren, you feel so good because, for an instant, you have tricked your mind into thinking you are a child. Do it more and get more of that feeling more of the time, and you can make yourself younger

Khalil Gibran (1883–1931) wrote about children and said, 'You may strive to be like them [your children] but seek not to make them like you.' If your husband is playing with the train set or flying his son's or grandson's kite, don't laugh at him, laugh *with* him, or play on a pogo stick or trampoline together and feel young. When you stop, notice that tingling sensation all over your body – it is the life force, the energy of your cells feeling revitalised and young.

FIND TIME FOR PLAY

Having been a single parent, I am aware that sometimes you just feel too stressed or overworked to play, and I've been to enough parties where the hosts feel they are too busy making the party a success to play. You don't have to engage in childlike things all the time, but just do it some of the time on a regular basis. You need only to take a few minutes to enjoy yourselves too, especially since it will result in you looking and feeling younger. At my daughter's first birthday party I was so busy doing things that I forgot to take one single photograph of the happy day, and since then I have made a point of enjoying myself each year.

I also went to a good friend's wedding and found her in tears. She was so busy trying to make everything just right and perfect for everyone else that she felt it was not her day any longer and she was not having fun at all. On what was meant to be one of the happiest days of her life she was feeling stressed, tense and miserable. I have done that in the past. I have spent so long organising a party or dinner and then not enjoyed it. I've not had fun, but that was the whole point of giving the party in the first place.

To stay young, do new things, because monotony ages anyone and variety is the spice of life. People who are young always look forward to something, and they also look forward to new things; they must have heard the expression, 'When hope dies old age runs to meet you.'

It's never too late to be young and childlike, and never too late to have a happy childhood. If you did not do these things as a child, that is even more of a reason to do them now. Women like Felicity Kendall, Sally Field, Lulu and Goldie Hawn are good examples of being childlike and remaining young. They all share that young, girlish attitude, the giggle and body language of a child, which actually keeps them young. Even Barbara Cartland believed she was young, and she dressed and acted in a very girly way, which had a very positive effect on her. She lived until she was 98 and was a prolific writer, selling over a million novels and writing up until her death.

Rejuvenate your brain

You have the power to make your body become younger. You also have the power to make your mind become younger and to stay mentally young throughout your life. The brain is a self-rejuvenating organ but, like the body, it has to be used regularly in order to work to its best. By regularly stimulating your brain you can maintain mental agility into your nineties and beyond.

Just as you need to exercise your body to maintain its strength and agility, you need to keep doing mental exercise to stay young. Tests on university professors who were aged 60–74 years old found that they were as accurate on memory and mental tests as people much younger, and far better than many who shared their age because they had stayed intellectually active.

Your brain changes every day – even as you read this sentence parts of your brain are making changes in themselves. You can improve all your mental faculties by changing it more. When you create new connections, your brain becomes stronger. Your neurons (nerve cells) become more active and your brain is able to create new neural pathways. Scientists have learned that the brain generates new neurons throughout life, and that physical movement changes thoughts. Doing new things and engaging in neurobics (mental exercises that build new pathways in the brain) can grow the part of the brain called the hippocampus – which has a huge effect on memory and brain power. The more you learn things and memorise things the more connections are created and strengthened. Just brushing your teeth using the other hand, or using your phone or remote control in the other hand, and going upstairs using the other foot first, are the kind of neurobics that strengthen the brain and improve memory and mental agility.

Moses Chao, a professor of neuroscience and psychiatry at New York University School of Medicine, found that using the 'wrong' hand can boost production of brain-derived neurotrophic factor (BDNF), a protein that encourages the growth of nerve cells linked to long-term memory. When we're stressed, our BDNF production plummets, but when we do something different, it increases. Using new technologies like Google, Skype, Facebook and Twitter will stimulate brain circuitry and exercise the brain more than reading a book, because they are new activities. If you love reading, simply reading online and becoming familiar with news apps that you can read on smartphones and tablets will boost your brain power and keep you young because they are new and different.

Tests on animals that were kept mentally stimulated show that the neurons in their brains remained strong and continued to renew themselves, whereas when the same animals were not kept in stimulating surroundings the neurons withered. When you use your mind, the neurons become stronger and they lengthen, whereas without use the same neurons wither, shrivel and weaken.

GIVE YOUR BRAIN THE EXERCISE IT THRIVES ON

Your brain is a thinking organ that grows, whatever your age, by interacting with the world through perception and action. Mental stimulation improves brain function and protects against mental decline, as does physical exercise. Your brain is able to rewire itself even in old age and it can grow new neurons if you keep using it. Many age-related losses in memory or motor skills are as a result of inactivity, and a lack of mental exercise and stimulation. The brain is rather brutal in its use-it-or-lose-it action, so as long as you keep using your brain you are more likely to hold on to excellent mental abilities. If you continue to work your brain by participating in any of the following activities you will use and stretch your mental faculties. Practise and skill will keep your mind young, and this too will influence your body to remain young.

Mental exercises to keep your brain in good shape and your mind young include:

- Crossword puzzles and sudoku.
- Reading and keeping up with current affairs.
- Playing chess, draughts or word puzzles (if you use a smartphone to do the above the effects are even better).
- Memorising poems, facts and articles.
- Joining in radio and television quiz shows, competing with the contestants to answer questions, and participating in magazine and newspaper competitions, brain teasers and other mind activities.

- Learning something new, such as a new language or learning to play a musical instrument; performing in amateur dramatics and learning lines will all keep you mentally young.
- Using Google, Skype, Twitter, Facebook and a smartphone or tablet.
- Gluing colours, shapes, letters and numbers onto a tennis ball and calling them out as you bounce it off the wall or floor.
- You can even train your eyes to work better and to stay younger by beading or threading a string.

DON'T BE AN OLD THINKER

You need to embrace young thinking as well as young activities. Old thinkers won't dance around to music or skip down the road with the children or grandchildren in case the neighbours see them and think they are silly. Old thinkers won't go swimming because they don't like their body. They won't go to the gym or join exercise classes because they think that the other people there will be fitter and more attractive than them and they hate how they look in exercise apparel. They won't even consider skipping or riding a bike or playing a board game, because they see that as kid's stuff, and they have far more important things to do like cleaning the house, doing the laundry and getting ready for work. When the children are being silly and childlike and noisy, without thinking an old thinker will say, 'Stop being childish – act your age!'

Young thinkers, on the other hand, will join in the silliness and be childlike too. I heard myself saying to my daughter, 'Stop being a baby' when she was only 12 months old. I remember thinking, 'Why am I saying that she is a baby? She is allowed to be a baby.' Luckily, I have learned so much since then and have such a different awareness now, and I don't do that anymore.

Young thinkers on reading the report about rebounders reducing wrinkles and bags under the eyes would be buying one straight away. They wouldn't stop to think, 'I haven't got anywhere to put it', 'It will spoil my bedroom and I will feel embarrassed having to explain to my partner what it is for.' They might even use the rebounder in the garden – far from caring what the neighbours think, they would be telling everyone about this new and wonderful way of looking and feeling younger, and perhaps even inviting them to try it out. They would do rebounding with the children and act more like the children instead of wanting to make the children act like them.

One of my patients became so committed to exercising that he ran when it was dark, either at dusk or early in the morning, because he was severely overweight and did not want to be seen. But he was determined to exercise, so he found a way and, as he lost weight and changed shape, he then began to exercise with other people and eventually joined a class.

Exercise 10: Do youthful things

1   Using everything you have learned in this step, make a list in your notebook of all the things you are going to do that will make you feel younger and make your body become younger. These will be things that appeal to you that you will want to do and will be able to do. Decide when you are going to do them, and make sure you set aside the time and then commit to keeping to it. Make a playlist of your favourite songs and play it when you are doing the physical exercises. Play it in your car too, so that it becomes an anchor for lifting your spirits and

▶

reminding you that you are as young as you choose to feel at any given moment. Remember the words and keep singing them to yourself; songs can be so good for lifting your spirits and changing your state. That's why politicians use them at political rallies to such great effect and why boxers enter the ring to their favourite music.

2   From the list below, choose something you are going to embrace. By making newness and variety your friend, and routine your enemy, you will absolutely slow ageing down. Doing any of the ideas listed below will make you feel young. It doesn't matter if you feel slightly silly; that feeling will soon go, and the benefits to your cells will soon compensate you.

3   Put on some music from the past and allow yourself to dance to it.

4   Play some music with a message about youth and sing out loud to it.

5   Ride a bike or spend a few minutes jumping on a pogo stick.

6   Bounce on a rebounder.

7   Skip with a skipping rope.

8   Play some board or card games from your childhood.

9   Find something funny – an article, cartoon or film – and every day look at the section that makes you laugh. When you have become immune to it, find another.

▶

10 If you have friends who are funny, hang around with them more; giggle and laugh, and do childlike things on a frequent basis. Remember, one of the best sounds in the world is that of children laughing.

11 Watch a children's film, such as *Mary Poppins* or *Fantasia*, and enjoy watching it like a child again.

12 Recreate all the wonderful feelings you created when you first fell in love.

13 Observe how children are, and become more like them.

Find out how old your body is

Finally, here are some exercises that will establish your biological age and show you how old your body is. As you do these tests, it is important to remember that your organs age to their own timetable, therefore you need to mark yourself separately on each test and then work out an average to get your biological age. The test on page 114 gives you a second way to find your biological age. It is quite hard to work out an accurate biological age using standard tests, as most of them work out an average without taking into account that at least 13 different measurements need to be taken. With these tests, however, you will get a good idea of how you are ageing biologically, and you will notice your ageing is improving as you stick to this programme and re-test yourself again later. The aim of these tests is to give you a base-line measurement that you can go on to improve. If you discover your biological age is higher than your chronological age, don't despair; just stick to the programme and re-test yourself in a few weeks and you will find that your biological age is becoming younger.

Be sure to note down your score in your notebook so that you can compare it as you become younger.

Tests for your biological age

TEST FOR BALANCE

1 You are going to do this test with your eyes closed. Stand
   barefoot on the floor, keep both feet together and close
   your eyes. Lift your left foot if you are right handed, and
   your right foot if you are left handed. Lift your foot 15cm
   (6in) off the floor with your knee bent.
2 Time yourself to see the amount of time you can hold this
   position without either opening your eyes or lowering your
   foot. Do this three more times and work out your average
   score.

Seconds	Biological age
28	20–30
22	30–40
18	40–50
10	50–60
4	60–70

TEST FOR YOUR REACTIONS

1 Ask a friend to hold a 46cm (18in) ruler vertically in front
   of you within your reach with the 1cm (or 1in) mark at the
   top. Hold your hand underneath the ruler with your thumb
   and middle finger positioned 4cm (1½in) apart.

2 Ask your friend to drop the ruler, then catch it as quickly as
   you can and note the centimetre (inch) mark at which you
   catch it. Repeat another two times to get an average.

Inches	Biological Age
11 or more	20
9	30
8	40
7	50
6 or less	60+

TEST FOR SKIN ELASTICITY

1   Put your hand on a flat surface with your fingers splayed out. Now pinch the skin on the back of one hand with the thumb and index finger of your other hand, hold for five seconds and let go.
2   Now count the number of seconds it takes for the skin to return to its previous condition free of puckering and ridging.

Seconds	Biological age
Less than 1	20–30
Over 2	30–40
5 or less	under 50
6–10	under 60
10–21	over 60

NAIL TEST

1   Put one of your fingernails under a bright light and, looking at it close up and from all angles, notice the following:

Nail condition	Biological age
Clear, healthy nail	20–30
Slightly ridged	30–40
Obvious ridging	40–50
Dry with obvious ridging	50–60
Discoloured and very noticeable or extreme ridging	60+

TEST FOR FLEXIBILITY

1   Sit on the floor with your right leg stretched out ahead of you and the sole of your left foot placed against your inner right thigh. Now stretch your right arm as far as you can towards your toes and make a note of how far you can reach. Make sure you stretch from the waist, not the shoulders.

Flexibility	Biological age
Reaching past your toes with your fingers	20–30
Reaching your toes with your fingers	30–40
Reaching your ankle with your fingers	40–50
Reaching mid-calf with your fingers	60s

TEST FOR YOUR EYESIGHT

1   Hold a book or newspaper at arm's length, then bring the page towards you until the print blurs.
2   Now measure the distance between yourself and the page. According to your age and eyesight you should be able to see the words quite clearly from your arm's length to a distance of:

Inches	Biological age
13cm (5in) or less	20–25
15–25cm (6–10in)	26–30
20–33cm (8–13in)	30–40
25–38cm (10–15in)	40–50
33–64.5cm (13–25in)	50s
100cm (39in) or less	60s

Make a note of your scores in your notebook

CALCULATE YOUR BIOLOGICAL AGE

1   In your notebook, write down your chronological age.
Subtract and add to it as necessary using the lists below to
reach your biological age.

  a   If you exercise regularly, subtract 4
  b   If your exercise recovery rate is quick, subtract 1
  c   If you sleep easily and regularly, subtract 1
  d   If you have a healthy sex life, subtract 2
  e   If your endurance and breathing are good, subtract 1
  f   If you laugh a lot, subtract 2
  g   If you are optimistic by nature, subtract 2
  h   If your diet is healthy, subtract 2
  i   If you are overweight by more than 10 per cent, add 3
  j   If your diet is unhealthy, add 2
  k   If you have poor digestion, add 2
  l   If you smoke, add 2
  m   If you drink every day, add 1
  n   If you get depressed often, add 1
  o   If you often get ill, colds, aches and pains, add 1
  p   If you get breathless, add 1
  q   If you sunbathe frequently, add 2

Summary – Step Four

Let's recap what you learned in this step.

- By putting what you have learned into practice you can achieve a younger body and a younger mental state. In this step you have learned the importance of acting on a regular basis as if you were young. You have learned that when you do young things your body literally grows younger.
- You have learned that something as simple as laughing and giggling, singing and dancing, listening to happy music from the past or skipping and jumping can cause us to instantly regress back to our youth, not just with our thoughts but also with our bodies.
- You have learned how to test your biological age.
- You have learned how to keep your mind and body young.

'A man is only as old as the woman he feels'

Groucho Marx (1890–1977)

(... and of course a woman is only as old as the man she feels)

Follow the Rules of the Mind

'If you do what you've always done, you'll get what
you've always got'

Various

Understanding the rules of how your mind works will help you to
influence your mind positively, rather than being influenced by
thoughts, beliefs and behaviours that you do not want. Imagine
that you purchased a top-of-the-range computer or washing
machine and it came without instructions. How would you use it?
You might find that you could not use it at all, or you might
muddle through, but you would never get the best out of your
machine. You could never use it to its full capacity, and you
would not get the excellent results that it was capable of giving to
you. We come into this world with the most amazing computer-
like brain that is capable of doing so much, but there are no
instructions given that tell us how to get the best from ourselves,
and we have no manual that shows us how to program ourselves
for success. We muddle through, when we are capable of so much
more. You can find instructions on how to take charge of your
body, weight and shape, but very little on how to run your mind.
This is changing slowly, however, and there are some books and

courses available now that will point you in the right direction. Some of them are excellent, and I look forward to the day when this information is taught in schools.

Here is a list of the rules of the mind as they apply to ageing. By reading them you will have a greater understanding of yourself and how you can influence the way you age. Some of them may seem a little repetitive and cover information that you have already come across in the first three steps, but your mind learns by repetition and it locks on to things that it hears repeatedly, so see this repetition as a good thing.

The rules of the mind are . . .

RULE 1: EVERY THOUGHT OR IDEA CAUSES A PHYSICAL REACTION

Thoughts have consequences and create changes in the body. Your thoughts create chemical reactions in your body. I have explained throughout the first section of this book about thoughts having consequences and creating changes in the body, so you already know this rule.

Ideas that have a strong emotional content always reach the subconscious mind, because it is the feeling mind. Once accepted, these ideas create the same reactions in the body again and again. To change negative reactions in the body it is important to change the ideas responsible for the reaction, both consciously and subconsciously.

If you have strong negative emotions linked to ageing, they will move into your subconscious mind and have a very real effect on you. By changing your thoughts so that you have strong *positive* emotions linked to ageing you can ensure that the effect your thoughts and emotions have on your body is positive and beneficial.

RULE 2: WHAT IS EXPECTED TENDS TO BE REALISED

The brain and nervous system respond to mental images regardless of whether the image is real or imagined. The mental image formed becomes the blueprint, and the subconscious mind uses every means at its disposal to act according to the blueprint. Worrying about ageing is a form of programming a picture of what we don't want (the blueprint), but the subconscious mind acts to fulfil the picture it's seeing. That is why it's so important not to create or hold on to pictures in your mind about the negatives connected to ageing but to decide instead to defy, challenge and redefine ageing. Our physical health can be absolutely linked to our mental expectancy. If we say, 'I'm bound to get a cold, because I got caught in the rain or put on damp clothes', then we usually will. Instead of expecting a decline into poor health as you get older, remove every despondent and negative attitude about ageing and expect to age fabulously. Expect to maintain health, strength and a feeling of well-being. Expect to continue to look and feel great with a sharp mind and these expectations will be realised.

RULE 3: IMAGINATION IS MORE POWERFUL THAN KNOWLEDGE WHEN DEALING WITH YOUR OWN MIND OR THE MIND OF ANOTHER

Reason is easily overruled by imagination. Violence would be unheard of if logic were able to override the emotional reaction. We can all stand on a piece of wood on the floor, but if that piece of wood became a plank placed high up between two buildings, the image of us falling would become more powerful than the knowledge that we can stand there if we have to. Any idea accompanied by a strong emotion, such as anger, fear, jealousy or panic, is more powerful than any logical information meant to disprove it. Your imagination and your ability to see yourself as younger, to believe you can slow down ageing, is more powerful than any medical data that says it can't be done. Science now says it can be done, and there is well-documented proof of examples of age reversal, so you really have no reason to age prematurely when there are so many things you can do to ensure you age excellently.

RULE 4: EACH SUGGESTION ACTED UPON CREATES LESS OPPOSITION TO SUCCESSIVE SUGGESTIONS

Once a suggestion has been accepted by the subconscious mind it becomes easier for additional suggestions to be accepted and acted upon. If we assume that this book has already caused you to accept some new suggestions, you can take faith in the knowledge that this alone is making it easier for you and for your mind to accept further beneficial information about staying young.

RULE 5: AN EMOTIONALLY INDUCED SYMPTOM TENDS TO CAUSE ORGANIC CHANGES IF PERSISTED WITH FOR LONG ENOUGH

Many doctors have acknowledged that more than 75 per cent of human ailments are functional rather than organic, meaning that the function of an organ or other body part has been disturbed by the nervous system's reaction to negative ideas held in the subconscious mind. We cannot separate the mind from the body, so if you dread ageing and constantly focus on getting old, on feeling and looking older, if you are searching for new wrinkles and looking for grey hairs, then in time negative organic changes must occur. If you believe that you can control how you age and keep your mental faculties, and maintain energy and agility while looking young, then positive organic changes are much more likely to occur.

RULE 6: WHEN DEALING WITH THE SUBCONSCIOUS MIND AND ITS FUNCTIONS, THE GREATER THE CONSCIOUS EFFORT, THE LESS THE SUBCONSCIOUS RESPONSE

Will power is not the tool to use when implementing change. Haven't we all tried to remember something, tried really hard and yet haven't remembered it, and then found that once we stopped trying the information we are looking for springs to mind? This is because the more conscious effort you make, the less the subconscious responds. Trying to go to sleep doesn't work for an insomniac, and trying to relax is ineffective for anxious people.

When you are making physical changes by using exercise, it's true that the more effort you put in the more results you will get back, but when you are making mental changes – when you are changing your thoughts, beliefs and expectations – the opposite applies. You don't need to try, you just need to let your subconscious absorb these new ideas. Let your mind accept them by being open to them. When making mental changes, effort is not truly necessary; what is necessary is the ability to get an image of how you plan to be (young, youthful, healthy, and mentally and physically fit) and to hold that image in your mind. Relax into the image and use language that matches the image. Keep re-running the image so that you are rehearsing it to such an extent that your brain thinks, 'I have been here before. I know how to do this – it's easy.'

As you take on new beliefs about ageing, you will replace all the old negative ones, but you must do it fully and program your subconscious mind specifically. So, form good images about ageing in your subconscious mind – the feeling mind – which is able to remove, alter or amend older negative ideas and beliefs.

RULE 7: ONCE AN IDEA HAS BEEN ACCEPTED BY THE SUBCONSCIOUS MIND, IT REMAINS THERE UNTIL IT IS REPLACED BY ANOTHER IDEA

The companion rule to this is:

RULE 8: THE LONGER THE IDEA REMAINS, THE MORE
OPPOSITION THERE IS TO REPLACING IT WITH A NEW IDEA

Once an idea has been accepted, it tends to remain. The longer it is held the more it tends to become a fixed way of thinking. This is how habits of action are formed both good and bad. First is the habit of thought, and then the habit of action. We have habits of thinking as well as habits of action, but the thought or idea always comes first. Therefore, if we want to change our actions we must begin by changing our thoughts. The poet John Dryden (1631–1700) said, 'We first make our habits and then our habits make us.'

We have many thought habits that are incorrect but are still fixed in the mind. Some people believe that at critical times they must have a drink to steady their nerves or a tranquilliser to calm them down. This is not necessarily true. The tranquilliser they take could even be a placebo, but the idea is there, and it is a fixed habit of thought. There can be opposition to replacing it with a correct idea. These are fixed ideas, not fleeting thoughts, but no matter how fixed the ideas are, or how long they have been held, they can absolutely be changed.

All beliefs, even very strong beliefs, can be changed if you introduce doubt, as we saw in Step Two, because the minute you begin to question something you no longer really believe it. If you ask someone if their partner is faithful, they will have a belief or a conviction, but if you suggest to them that you know otherwise, that you have information that their partner is seeing someone else, you might place doubt in their mind. It very much depends on their belief system. If you ask someone if they believe in God, most people who are religious are in no doubt and won't question their beliefs. Now look at all your beliefs about ageing and about how you expect to age. Are they negative beliefs or very positive ones? You will find all the information in this programme to allow you to introduce doubt into any negative belief, conviction or opinion about ageing.

RULE 9: THE MIND CANNOT HOLD CONFLICTING BELIEFS

The mind cannot hold conflicting thoughts either. We can't be honest and dishonest at the same time or happy and sad simultaneously. If you hold conflicting beliefs it sends the mind into a spin and blocks the mind from moving you towards what it is that you really want. Making lots of jokes about the supposed horrors of getting old, or exaggerating through jokes what we perceive as ageing, does this. We cannot plan to age well and then engage in joking about the awfulness of ageing, because the beliefs are contradictory. They confuse the mind, which has to take everything we say as the literal truth. I mentioned earlier that we are controlled by what we link pain and pleasure to. People who are successful in any area, such as relationships, health or career, have very clear definitions; for example, if you long to be in love but fear becoming vulnerable when this happens or that one day you might be rejected by your lover, then you are linking pleasure and pain to the same thing and the mind can't move towards pleasure and away from pain, because they are linked to the same thing – in this instance being in love. If you want to be hugely successful but you link pain to hard work or not having your weekends free, then you have mixed associations, which you must change. Pain is always the more dominant emotion and your mind will do more to avoid pain than it will to get pleasure, because avoiding pain is how we survive on the planet. Bulimics are an interesting example of mixed associations because they link pain and pleasure to food. They hate being full and yet love being full. They love food, but they detest even the smell of it. They usually think of food all day yet they want to be indifferent to food, often reading cookery books yet not wanting to eat.

Changing your associations makes life so much easier, and humans are the only creatures lucky enough to be able to choose what to associate pain or pleasure to. It has been said that the major advantage – and equally disadvantage – of humans is that they can choose what to link pain and pleasure to. I can choose to love eating meat or to link pain to it, and thus become a vegetarian, but I would find it hard if I linked pleasure to meat while deciding to give it up. If I hate exercising and link pain to it but feel I have to do it, it will always be a chore, but if I decide I want to exercise and that I will enjoy it, it becomes more of a pleasure.

Whatever changes you make as a result of reading this book, make sure you link pleasure to them. If you hate exercising, but make yourself do it, you will lose some of its benefits. If you give up junk food, but resent doing so, your mind will link pain to healthy eating and you might always feel deprived, instead of knowing that you have made some life-enhancing choices and are feeling great and proud about them.

When you make these choices, don't say 'I must', 'I have to', or 'I have got to'. Instead, say 'I want to' or 'I have chosen to'. It is such a simple change, and yet it makes such a big difference. When I was first writing this book, I had some resistance to spending my weekends writing. Friends would invite me over and I would say, 'I can't, I have to write my book', yet when I began to say 'I want to write this weekend' or 'I have chosen to spend this weekend writing' I felt entirely different and noticed that I was enjoying the process and really did not want to be anywhere else. I was amazed that on a wonderful sunny weekend I was so happy and content writing away, and in that moment there was nowhere else I wanted to be.

Around university examination time, I hypnotise a lot of students and I always tell them that they have *chosen* to study, that for this particular month they *want* to revise, and that it is *compelling*, they actually *enjoy* the process, and it makes them feel *so good* to do the work. They almost always send in friends who say, 'You hypnotised my friend to study, and it's amazing, he's actually enjoying it! Can you do the same for me please?'

If you make a point of linking massive pleasure to the changes you are making by filling up your mind with good thoughts, words and pictures, you will move towards the changes more easily. If you link huge amounts of pain to being inactive, or to smoking, you will move away from them more easily. Loving your body helps a lot, because the more you love your body the less you want to hurt it or abuse it. You are able to choose how you feel, so link pleasure to changing years, and don't link pain, despair or fear to getting older, or you will accelerate the process. You cannot plan to look, feel and become years younger while dreading ageing.

Exercise 11: Remove pain and substitute pleasure

For the written exercises in this section, I want you to use your imagination. Don't worry if you feel you don't have one. You do, you are just not aware of it.

1   Imagine your brain is like a computer screen divided into two columns headed 'pleasure' and 'pain'. Under the heading of 'pain' are negative pictures and words about ageing, whereas under the heading of 'pleasure' are positive images and words about ageing.

2   Now imagine making the 'pleasure' column bigger, brighter and more joyful, using images and words to create pictures of you looking and feeling good at every stage of your life. You then link pleasure to your ability to age in a way that suits you and inspires others as you become wiser and happier.

3   Now imagine yourself looking at the 'pain' section and seeing all the pain you have unconsciously linked to getting older, then delete this section completely, just as you would on a computer screen. Delete all the beliefs that only youth is good or desirable; see how ridiculous and untrue this belief is, and remind

▶

yourself that being young is not without its own problems (as we have seen, the highest suicide group in the world, for example, is young people and, especially, teenagers).

Your mind is programmed to move you towards pleasure and away from pain, and it will always do more to avoid pain than it will to seek pleasure. This is why many people won't risk talking to a stranger they are attracted to, or ask someone for help if they need it. The pain of possible rejection is more powerful than the pleasure they might gain. Moving away from pain is a survival instinct built into our system. From early in our evolution we have linked pain to things that hurt us and we have avoided them from that moment on. If you link pain to ageing, you will always hanker after youth and always feel disadvantaged. If you link pleasure to changing, and if you change your thoughts, you will change your reality and then you will be able to become and remain younger throughout your long and happy life.

Use affirmations to feel younger

Now you are familiar with the rules of the mind you are ready to go on to learn about affirmations and how to use them, which can really help you to look and feel younger.

Affirmations are statements of truth. An affirmation is simply a short statement you repeat to yourself over and over for a few minutes daily. It might be something like: 'I always look younger than my years', or 'My memory is as good as that of a 30-year-old', or 'I am becoming younger all the time', or 'I am taking the correct action that makes me look, feel and become younger', or

'I am a walking, talking expression and example of youthfulness.' You repeat the affirmation over and over, out loud to yourself, to allow your subconscious mind to accept it.

It won't always happen instantly, because we often pick an affirmation that can conflict with some beliefs we may have. One of the reasons we are covering affirmations at this point is because by now you will have changed some beliefs and will be open to the idea of changing more.

Many people give up with affirmations, because their mind seems to have so many objections to them. They don't really believe what they are saying, or they don't understand that there is a system for making the mind accept and believe affirmations, so they find the process frustrating and then abandon it.

I have found the best way to overcome this is to write out each affirmation in your notebook as a statement, and just notice any objections that come to mind. Then you write out the objections your mind comes up with. Keep on writing out the affirmation, with any objections or thoughts that come to mind written directly underneath the affirmation. It is important not to spend time attempting to analyse or rationalise the objections. Just write them out and keep going, so that you write down each affirmation and any objection or response. As you look over the statement and the objections you have written, you may notice a distinct pattern emerging, because the more you keep writing out the affirmation, the fewer objections your mind will come up with. Eventually your mind will exhaust the objections, and it will simply say, 'OK, I agree, I accept it. You are slowing down ageing.'

Here's an example, let's say your chosen affirmation is:

'I am *becoming* and *remaining* younger.'

Your mind may immediately come up with some objections, especially if you have been conditioned by the beliefs of others. These may be something like:

- You cannot become younger.
- It is not possible to become younger.
- How can anyone stay younger?
- I have never heard of anyone remaining younger.
- Everyone will laugh at me if I do this.
- This is all rubbish.
- I don't believe in this.

Then you will notice the objections soften, change and diminish as your mind comes up with:

- Actually, I do believe in this.
- There are examples of people growing younger.
- If other people can do it, so can I.
- OK, it's true, I can and will become younger.

As you continue to write out each affirmation and to say it out loud, your objections will become weaker and weaker, you will pay them less and less attention and your belief in your affirmation will become stronger. Eventually, your mind will run out of objections and it will then fully accept the affirmation.

Get into the habit of repeating your affirmations daily, and make sure you say them out loud. It doesn't matter if you feel silly; most people do initially. Just become aware of how you feel and the thoughts and feelings you experience as you say each affirmation. It's good to repeat your affirmations at night just before you go to sleep, and again in the morning just after waking, when your subconscious is at its most receptive. It is also a very good idea to write out your affirmations and to pin them up on a mirror or the fridge door, to put them in your purse or your desk, on your screen saver and on your phone, and anywhere else that prompts you to remind yourself of them regularly and frequently. By doing this you will be able to make your ability to stay younger an on-going affirmation.

YOUR AFFIRMATIONS AS A POSITIVE BLUEPRINT

You will develop more and more potential through the use of your affirmations, because the words and images you repeat over and over to yourself become the blueprint for who you become. Positive affirmations go into the subconscious and eventually replace negative thoughts. The subconscious responds best to clear, authoritative commands. The clearer, more precise and straightforward they are, the more rapidly the mind accepts them and begins to work on them.

Affirmations can also build self-esteem, turn you into an optimist, and diminish negative self-talk. Please make sure you write out your affirmations in your notebook using the instructions in this chapter. Write out every objection you come up with until you have exhausted them. Then look at what you have written and what you can learn and benefit from.

Summary – Step Five

Let's recap what you have learned in this step.

- You have learned all the rules of the mind and how they apply directly to how you are ageing.
- You have learned how to influence your mind so that what you link pain and pleasure to is up to date and works in your favour.
- You have learned how to make affirmations correctly so that they work for you.

'Man is made by his belief. As he believes, so he is'

Johann Wolfgang von Goethe (1749–1832)

How to Visualise Perfectly to Age Well

'What the mind of man can conceive and believe it can achieve'

Napoleon Hill (1883–1970)

In this step, I am going to show you how to easily and effectively program your mind to slow down ageing. In order to do this, you absolutely must be able to see yourself defying ageing, looking younger and feeling, thinking and acting younger. You can do it with practice, and if you take just five minutes every day to visualise yourself as youthful, and mentally and physically fit, you are raising your chances of becoming and staying that way. Scientists in the US and Europe have proved that visualisation techniques dramatically affect our bodies. When you see yourself as young and active, you send a clear message to your brain that affects your energy levels, your hormones, and your motivation. These changes cause physical sensations, which in turn affect your thoughts and feelings, and those in turn reinforce the mental programming. Thinking positively about ageing can activate particular neurons in the brain, which secrete hormones such as endogenous opiates, which make us feel good about ourselves. Negative thoughts have the opposite effect. Particular neurons are involved with producing negative thoughts, and they also produce negative hormones, such as cortisol, a stress hormone that leads to feelings of anxiety, which in itself is very ageing.

While forming different pictures in your mind, you must also eliminate every possible negative word and focus only on what you wish to achieve. Keep your mind on what you want, and off what you don't want. Whatever you focus on, you will move towards, so focusing on not ageing and not feeling old simply puts negative words and images back into your mind.

How to program the subconscious mind to age less

Today you are going to learn how to visualise perfectly. I can already hear you saying, 'I am no good at visualising. It just doesn't work for me, I don't have an imagination.' I know right now you believe that, but it is just not true. We all have an imagination or we would never worry, or respond to scary images on the television. I frequently meet clients who say things like, 'I can't imagine things' or 'I'm just no good at visualisation.' I say to them, 'That's great! You must never worry about anything – ever.'

'Oh, but I do,' they say.

And I respond, 'How can you worry if you can't imagine or visualise? How do you find your car when you return to the car park if you don't have an ability to visualise where you parked it hours earlier?'

You could never drive anywhere without a map or satnav unless you are able to visualise the route you take. It is impossible to worry unless you have an imagination and can visualise, so if you have ever worried about anything, you have a great imagination and you already possess wonderful visualisation skills.

Visualisation takes practice, and it gets easier, because what the mind sees, it believes without question. What you can hold in your mind you can accomplish, and as you visualise, you will stimulate your mind and body into action. Everyone has an imagination, and your imagination has no limits. If you think you can't see or imagine your body remaining young and your mind staying as sharp as a tack, remember the power of thought. Thinking of it will make it happen. When you think, or even hear, about something, your mind always makes a picture of what that looks like. Even though you believe you are not able to visualise, your mind is actually seeing it in great detail – you are just not aware of it. During this programme, when I describe cells becoming younger or healthier it really does not matter if you feel you can't *see* your cells becoming younger, just remember what I have told you about the amazing power of thought: *thinking of it will make it happen.* Your mind is actually seeing it in great detail, you are just not aware of it. You can see yourself as young, and you can see yourself staying young and even becoming younger. This book is showing you exactly how to achieve this. Everything that happens is linked to how we see ourselves. You can and will become younger to the degree that you are able to see yourself as youthful. When you practise skills of visualisation, and combine them with programming the subconscious mind, you will get very definite results.

INSTRUCT YOUR CELLS THROUGH THOUGHT

We have amazing potential to influence our cells, to tell them how to behave, and to make them act accordingly. I always describe cells as being like a class of young children. They know exactly what to do and how to do it, but if they aren't working to our satisfaction – or, in the case of cells, if they have started to break down or malfunction – they need to be commanded, instructed or shown what to do using the power of thought, visualisation and imagination. You won't believe it when you see it, but you will see it when you believe it.

What we see and believe is what we ultimately become. Step Nine of this programme goes into this in more detail and uses the power of thought and imagination by using prepared scripts to direct cells to act as younger cells do. Your mind already has a memory of how your body performed when you were at your peak, and you can manifest this just by thinking of it. This means that as you think about cells performing in a particular way, you can activate their ability to perform in that way.

Think hard about swallowing. Do it now, as you read this, and you will notice that you want to swallow. Your mind responds to the picture and makes you do it. Think about blinking, and you will find yourself blinking, because what we think about, the body brings about. This happens both consciously and subconsciously. After thinking about looking younger and reading or listening to the scripts for a few days, you will find the words and descriptions become embedded in your mind and you can relate and refer to them easily and automatically. This will have an effect on your skin, collagen and elastin, your organs and on your sense of well-being. Even as you sleep, your subconscious mind is affecting your hormones, increasing blood flow, affecting your skin and skin cells, and also your muscles, which have a memory all of their own.

THE POWER OF THE SUBCONSCIOUS

Your subconscious mind is much stronger than your conscious mind. It is said that only 10 per cent of our mind is conscious and the other 90 per cent is subconscious, and that willpower accounts for only 4 per cent of the conscious-mind percentage. The conscious mind is the mind of choice, whereas the subconscious is the mind of preference, and we always choose what we prefer. In areas of conflict, the subconscious mind will always win, because it can make the conscious do whatever it likes. This is particularly relevant in areas such as overeating, where the conscious desire may be to lose weight, but the subconscious has some deeper preference for the excess weight, often as a form of insulation or barrier. The subconscious desire is more likely to win, because it is more dominant and able to affect the workings of your body.

Some hypochondriacs have a strong conscious desire to be well, but the subconscious desire is to be ill, because illness allows them to receive attention, including love, touch, nurturing, time and concern. Although they may wish to be well, they also have a subconscious desire to be ill which is more dominant. The subconscious is at least 90 per cent stronger than the conscious, and the subconscious mind works 30,000 times faster than the conscious. If you are set on making changes but you think you have only to make them consciously, you will find it a harder, longer, less successful and a less lasting process than if you make those changes subconsciously.

If you want to change any behaviour, you must be absolutely sure to make changes both consciously and subconsciously. Your mind will always do what it thinks you want it to do, but unless you are clear when programming your mind it will do things with the right intention but often get the wrong result. It is rather like finding that someone who came in to clean your house has moved all your things and put them back in the wrong place. That person's intention is to help you, but unless you are able to clearly state, 'Don't move the papers on my desk, and don't throw out that pile of magazines, but please do this and this', you won't get the result you intended. You would have got a better result if you had been clearer and more detailed in your instructions. If you go to the hairdresser and say, 'Cut my hair', without being specific, it is not very likely that you will get the cut you want, even though the hairdresser is doing what he or she thinks you want. It is the same with your mind. If you are detailed and specific, you are more likely to get what you want, but if you are vague and unspecific, you are less likely to get what you want.

Specificity is important because your mind has no capacity to reason. It will lock on to ideas that are not specific or detailed enough or are outdated, and you won't get the results you want or could have. Your subconscious mind has only one job to do and that is to move you towards pleasure and away from pain and to do what it thinks you want it to; for example, if someone longed for attention, he could develop a nervous habit, which would get him lots of attention, but not the kind he wanted. If you want attention, make sure you programme your subconscious by letting it know that you want only positive, beneficial attention. When children want attention, they don't care if it's positive or negative. They just want attention. Some children and adults can fall victim to a variety of illnesses, because they are not getting the attention they need.

Sometimes the subconscious need or desire for attention can be so great that it can cause a person to go from one symptom of illness to another, completely overruling the conscious desire to be fit and well.

If you long for a rest because you are overworked, and say things like, 'I would love a week off, just staying in bed', and then you end up in bed with flu, it is an example of the subconscious being incorrectly programmed. If you say that you are dreading the party or meeting on Wednesday and that you would give anything not to go, you might wake up on Wednesday with an upset stomach or severe headache that prevents you from going. Your mind thinks it has done what you wanted and, in a way, it has, but in a very ineffective and counterproductive way.

I once worked with a girl who was late for everything, causing her lots of anxiety and unhappiness. She realised, while in hypnosis, that this started as a child when she was desperate for attention and would miss the school bus so that her father would have to drive her to school. As an adult, she was continuing the pattern of being late, and was attracting lots of unwanted attention, because she was a teacher and would always be the last to arrive at her own class. When she'd attend a lecture or concert, she would always be the last one to enter the room, so everyone would turn to look at her, or stand up to let her pass, which she hated but it got her a lot of attention. She was able to change this behaviour by letting her subconscious know that this practice was outdated and inappropriate, that it caused her anxiety and had a negative effect on her career. Having told herself that she only wanted positive and beneficial attention, she ceased being late and actually started to get to places early. She was delighted with this, because it made such a difference in her life. She was calmer, she did not miss trains or appointments, and she was able to develop a reputation for being punctual (although it took her friends and family a while to get used to the new behaviour).

YOU CAN BE AN EXPERT

It is such an asset to understand how the subconscious works. Once you learn how to programme your mind to your advantage, you will see that your mind is a great and powerful ally. It will do what you ask it or tell it to do, if you ask in a specific way. Your mind is the most effective and powerful tool for implementing positive changes in your life. As you follow each chapter of this book, step by step, you will become an expert at programming your subconscious mind, and you will find that the more you do it, the better you will become at it, and the more you will enjoy it.

The steps to programming the subconscious mind for ageless ageing

1 BE POSITIVE

Eliminate every possible negative word connected to ageing, and focus only on what you wish to achieve – ageless ageing – and move towards it. Don't focus on the opposite, which is what you wish to leave behind.

2 BE *ABSOLUTELY* CLEAR

Keep your mind *on* what you want and *off* what you don't want. Whatever you focus on, you will move towards, so thinking about how you don't want to look or feel or become simply puts negative words and images of how you don't want to be back into your mind. For example, 'I feel excited and positive about every stage of my life', not 'I am not scared about getting older'; 'I am looking and feeling younger all the time', not 'I don't look old and I don't feel old'; 'My energy level is great, I have abundant energy', not 'I no longer feel as tired as I used to'.

'No', 'not' and 'don't' are all neutral words and have no effect on the subconscious mind. That's why thinking the words 'I am not sleepy', 'I don't feel tired', causes the mind to lock on to the only descriptive words in the sentence which are 'tired' and 'sleepy'. If you keep saying 'I don't feel old' your mind is locking on to the descriptive word 'old', so replace it with 'I feel wonderfully healthy'. Thinking 'I am not getting older' focuses on the only descriptive word, which is 'older', so replace it with, 'I feel young, I am an expression of youthfulness.'

By turning over any negative thoughts, you will find the positive, because they are the flip side of your thinking.

One of my clients told me as soon as I met him, 'This hypnosis doesn't work, you know, because I read a book on how to hypnotise yourself and every night for weeks I would put myself into hypnosis and then tell myself I am not inadequate, I am not scared of people, I no longer feel stupid or tongue tied. It didn't work at all. I still feel inadequate.' I had to explain to him that his intentions were right but his programming was wrong, and once he learned how to communicate a different scenario to himself he began to get the results he wanted.

3 BE SPECIFIC – USE VERY DESCRIPTIVE WORDS

As I pointed out earlier, the words we use in front of words increase or decrease the effect of those words.

Rather than saying 'I feel healthy', say 'I feel *extremely* healthy' or '*fantastically* healthy'. Say 'I have abundant energy' or '. . . massive amounts of energy'. Instead of saying 'I like exercise', change it to 'I am passionate about exercise and feel invigorated after every gym visit.'

The mind only responds to words that are symbolic and which make a picture, so use words that are very symbolic and very descriptive; for example, 'I have smooth, satiny skin', 'I am flexible, supple and agile', 'I enjoy vigorous health', 'I have tremendous stamina', 'I look and feel marvellous', 'I have perfect cell regeneration.'

Don't worry if this all seems a little far-fetched and not strictly true. Your subconscious mind has no capacity to reason and will believe whatever you tell it, especially if you tell it often enough, so you might as well go for it and exaggerate every point.

In the English language there are 4,000 words for emotions and feelings yet, as we have seen, many people use the same 12 words over and over to describe how they are feeling – words like 'not bad', 'pretty good', 'OK', 'all right'. Using different words will change your biochemistry, so when you are describing yourself use words like 'magnificent', 'amazing', 'fabulous', 'excellent', 'phenomenal', 'superb', 'enthusiastic', 'exceptional', 'dynamic', 'marvellous', 'wonderful' and 'outstanding'.

4 USE THE PRESENT TENSE

The subconscious mind is only in the moment, so create images that are occurring now, this instant; for example, 'My skin is becoming more clear, healthy and attractive every day', 'This programme is working on me rapidly and progressively right now.'

Never use the word 'my' as a prefix to something you wish to be free from, such as 'My migraines', 'My wrinkles', 'My tired legs', 'My addiction', 'My aches and pains', 'My terrible memory'. This is making the mind accept something as belonging to you – which it doesn't. A good rule of thumb is this: if you don't want to keep it, don't call it 'mine'. Your mind finds it much easier to change things and let go of things when it believes you don't want them, but if you call those same things 'mine' it is very confusing to the mind. Remember that the mind cannot hold conflicting beliefs, so referring to something as 'mine' while wanting to be free of it is conflicting. It soon becomes easy and habitual to say 'the headache', 'the worries', 'the wrinkles'. Start doing it now and keep doing it. If you have a pain, instead of saying 'my aches and pains', or 'my indigestion', change it to 'the pain' and 'the poor digestion'.

If your programming says 'next year', or even 'next month I will look and feel younger', your mind cannot make a proper image of it, because your mind only works in the present tense, so you must say, 'I look younger now.' It is very beneficial to add the words 'now' or 'right now' to the end of every statement you make:

- My cells are repairing and replacing themselves perfectly right now.
- I am looking, feeling and becoming younger now.
- I am absorbing and benefiting from my vitamins right now.

5 BE DETAILED

Make your words dynamic and descriptive, such as, 'I am young, vibrant and full of life.' Make your statements personal: 'I am ...', 'I look ...', 'I always ...', 'I can ...'

6 YOUR VISUALISATION MUST BE *VIVID*

See your visualisation – sense it, feel it, touch it and hear it. Activate all your senses, because the more vividly you visualise the more rapidly your mind responds. See yourself as young, feel yourself enjoying excellent health, imagine touching your skin and feeling how soft and satiny it is. Sense your body responding to your instructions so that every cell is in the right place at the right time doing its work perfectly. Hear people commenting on how well and how young you look.

7 YOUR VISUALISATION MUST BE *FREQUENT*

The more vividly you visualise, the more rapidly your mind and body will respond. Visualise frequently, and repeat it over and over, like playing a film in your head. Repetition is vital. When you repeat an action, you create a neural pathway in your brain that is strengthened with each repetition. This pathway is like a thread that becomes stronger every time you repeat something, until it becomes more like a cable. When you first learned to use a keyboard, drive a car or operate a new mobile phone, you had to repeat the actions slowly. Now, due to repetition, they are so embedded in your mind and body that they are almost automatic.

8 USE DURATION AND INTENSITY

Hold the picture for longer and make it bigger, brighter and clearer. Combine your visualisation with an intensity of desire, as this will increase its effectiveness. Visualisation takes practice. What the mind sees it believes without question, so your ability to visualise will have a powerful effect on you. As you visualise, you will stimulate your mind and body into action. Remember: what you can hold in your mind with confidence and feeling, you can achieve.

Become much clearer about what you want. The more you visualise, the more you will believe your visualisation is possible. Successful people visualise all the time. We can all change our thinking and the mental pictures we make. As we improve them we can improve everything. By changing your thinking and your focus, and by making changes in the language you use, you can change your looks and your health forever. If you think you can't do it, be aware that you are already visualising that outcome all the time. Every time you say, 'I can't slow down ageing. It does not work for me', you are already visualising a specific result, and it's working. You might as well use good visualisations, as your mind will believe and act on whatever you tell it – whether good or bad – because your mind responds to the pictures you make in your head and the words you say to yourself.

Exercise 12: Your programme for becoming younger

You are now ready to make a programme specifically for you. Go through the following eight steps, and write it out as a plan. By step eight your thoughts will have developed into one or more paragraphs. Begin now by taking a thought, such as 'I am becoming younger', and write this out as number 1.

1   'I am becoming younger.'

2   For step 2, decide how you can be absolutely crystal clear about fact number 1, and write it out.

3   Now increase your sentence into a paragraph, using very descriptive words and keeping it all in the present tense. 'I am becoming younger by . . .' or 'I am becoming younger because . . .', or 'I am becoming younger as I . . .'

▶

4   Make it even more personal. This is all about *you* as you want to be, so add more words and thoughts. Put powerful positive words in front of your sentences, so increase it to 'I am becoming amazingly younger', 'I am a superb and excellent example of youth and vitality.' 'My body is . . .', 'I have the energy level of . . . ', and so on. Use several thoughts, and then connect them in a statement as you work through this exercise. The end result will leave you with an exciting, easy-to-memorise statement about yourself rather than several lines of short sentences.

5   Make it even more detailed by adding: 'I am . . .', 'I always . . .', 'I feel . . .', 'I can . . .', 'I look . . .', 'I have . . .' to your programme.

6   Use and activate all your senses by adding the words 'feel', 'sense', 'touch', 'see', 'hear', 'imagine'.

7   Keep working on it until you have it exactly as you want it, then read it and repeat it to yourself over and over until it becomes embedded in your mind. This will happen quite quickly and easily. Your programme should not be so long that you can't recall it, or so short that it does not make enough impact on your mind.

8   Now you are ready to close your eyes and begin to imagine what you have created and chosen for yourself. It really doesn't matter if you don't seem to make vivid pictures. By now your mind is absolutely responding to the words and images whether you are seeing them clearly or not.

▶

A finished example of this could be:

'I am becoming younger, my body is growing younger and my mind is always young. I know this to be true, because I think young thoughts and because I feel so young. I feel as healthy and as young as I felt in my teens. In fact I feel happier and more content, and I continue to look forward to every stage of my life. I am becoming younger by thinking young thoughts always. I am becoming younger because I have a belief system that allows me to believe and know this is possible. I am becoming younger because I have such a strong desire and belief in my ability to become and stay young.'

or

'I am a wonderful example of the power of the mind to slow ageing. I impress and inspire people I come into contact with because I am such an expression of youth. My body looks and feels young. I have abundant energy. I love the challenge of new things. I feel young because I believe I am young. I constantly hear people telling me how young and vibrant I am. My skin feels young and healthy, and I know my cells are forever young and healthy.'

Prepare well for excellent results

When we hold a thought, plan, goal or idea continuously in our mind, our subconscious works to bring it to reality. Many of my clients tell me that they don't believe this, because they have a plan in their minds that has never come to fruition. This is always because they have not done the groundwork, they have not cleared their mind of conflicting thoughts and beliefs beforehand. Although they may have a plan in their minds, they have not programmed their minds in a specific way that will allow the plan to be realised.

If you follow the detailed and specific steps designed to allow you to program your mind for success, you can succeed. You can continue to hold your programme in your mind by writing and rewriting it, reviewing it, talking about it and visualising it.

Some people are very visual and respond to how things look, whereas others respond better to how things sound or feel. This is known as being auditory, visual or kinaesthetic. Whichever you are, or whichever you predominantly are, this programme has been designed to work for you.

What kind of responder are you?

People who respond most instinctively to how things look are known as *visual*. People who respond to how things feel are known as *kinaesthetic* and people who respond to how things sound are known as *auditory*. It is possible to be a combination of all three or to be predominantly one with aspects of the others.

If you know that you are mostly visual, focus more of your programme on how you look, what your skin looks like, how young your body is and how good your vision is.

If you are more kinaesthetic, focus more on how you feel and what your skin and body feels like.

If you are predominantly auditory, you can focus on hearing everyone tell you how well you look.

You will find you can remember the programme by reading it at night before you go to sleep. It will quickly become embedded in your mind this way. It is also worth writing out the programme and reading it on your computer and phone. You can pin it onto your fridge or your mirror, and if you make a collage or poster, add your programme to that.

Summary – Step Six

Congratulations on all the work you have done. Let's recap what you have learned in this step.

- How to program your subconscious mind for success.
- How to visualise perfectly, even if you are not a very visual person.
- How to make a personal programme for yourself that you can believe in and that will excite your imagination. As you focus on this programme you will move towards its realisation.

'As you think so you are, as you continue to think so you remain'

Anonymous

Goals and Goal-setting for Ageing Well

'There is a fountain of youth: it is your mind, your talents, the creativity you bring in your life and the lives of people you love'

Sophia Loren

Now that you are becoming so good at making changes in yourself you are ready to understand the power of goals and to become a successful goal setter in the area of looking and feeling years younger. Many tests over many years, including several done at Harvard, Yale and Cornell universities, as well as the famous Maslow tests, show that people who set goals are always the happiest and have a very high tendency to achieve their goals.

Pinpointing your goals

Think about your goals. When you bought this book, you had a specific goal, which was to look and feel years younger. At this stage in the book, you have already made some changes that have increased your ability to achieve that goal.

Start to think now of the goals you would like to achieve for yourself in the area of ageing.

- How do you want to look ten years from now?
- How do you want to feel?
- What do you want to be doing with your life in the future?
- How do you plan to spend all these extra years since you are intending to live longer and remain active?

Make sure you have a goal that draws you forward into the future.

WRITE OUT YOUR GOALS

Having a goal, and taking steps to accomplish it, seems to fire within us a stronger ability to reach that goal. In 1979, members of the MBA graduating programme at Harvard were asked, 'Have you set clear, written goals for your future and made plans to accomplish them?' Only 3 per cent had done so; 13 per cent had goals that were not written out; and 84 per cent had no goals at all. Ten years later, the class was interviewed again. The results showed that the 3 per cent who had clear, written goals were earning ten times as much as the other 97 per cent were earning collectively. Even the 13 per cent who had unwritten goals were earning twice as much as the 84 per cent who had no goals. That Harvard study was a copy of a study done in 1953 at Yale University, where the graduating year was asked a series of questions, including, 'Do you have clear, specific goals written out, with plans to accomplish them?' Just 3 per cent said yes. Twenty years later, they went back and interviewed the class members again and found that the 3 per cent with written goals were worth more financially than the other 97 per cent put together. Not only were they dramatically richer but they were also happier, better adjusted and more successful at everything they did. That is the incredible power of habitually and systematically setting goals. You must write out your goals, think about your goals, talk about your goals, and make plans to achieve them, so your subconscious mind works to make your goals come to fruition. Current studies still show that less than 3 per cent of people have clear goals, and less than 1 per cent ever write them out correctly.

By setting anti-ageing goals you will become a member of an elite group, since less than 3 per cent of the population have any goals to become younger, or even know that such a thing is possible. This belief, however, is changing. One of my incentives in writing this book is to cause that low percentage to rise. As society begins to notice more and more people who are ageing fabulously – and it realises this isn't down to luck or a fluke, or even good genes, but because those people are taking the right actions and making the right choices to become younger – more people will follow suit. Having good genes will usually add only about three years to your life; having parents who both lived long lives won't add more than a few years to your own lifespan; but making lifestyle changes, and changing habits of thought and beliefs, can add 30 years or more to your life.

If you want to stay young, write it out as a goal in the specific format contained further along in this Step. When you programme your goals into your brain, you move towards accomplishing them much more easily. Of course, you need to do more than simply write out your goals as if they were a wish list. You need self-discipline, determination and the self-belief to stay with them until you accomplish them. Louis Pasteur (1822–95) said, 'Let me tell you the secret that has led me to my goal: my strength today lies solely in my tenacity.'

Understand that goal-setting points to success

It's hard to understand why more people aren't encouraged to set goals and why it is not taught in schools, especially since schools that have experimented with goal-setting find that children like it and benefit hugely from it. People don't set goals because they don't understand their importance. They don't know how to set goals because goal-setting is not taught in schools. They fear rejection, ridicule or criticism, so they hold back from goal-setting. They might fear failure without understanding that often you can't succeed without first encountering failure, as failing to get something correct the first time is how we learn. Almost all inventors encounter failure during the inventing process. The only way you can fail at anything is by failing to try.

As you write out your goals and write out your plan for reaching these goals, you are already taking action that moves you closer to achieving them, because your mind works in such a way that whatever you focus on, you move towards. Your subconscious mind is a natural goal-seeking device programmed to move you towards what it is you are focusing on. By focusing on your goals (especially as you write them out) you cannot help but activate the mechanism within yourself that moves you towards achieving them, because goals seem to trigger the success mechanism within us.

Simply having a goal to live longer and making plans to achieve that goal can make it happen. If you have a goal to become and remain younger and you put that goal into action, and you then make plans to achieve that goal, you will be successful. Medical tests have shown that people who have a goal to stay alive can even defy death, and numerous patients who have been close to death have literally postponed death until an important event, such as a birthday, a daughter's wedding, a birth in the family, or another significant date has passed. They have a goal to live until then, and tend to reach that goal. In China they have an annual day when elders are celebrated. It's a big event that older people look forward to the way children look forward to Christmas. More elderly people die directly after this date than at any other time of year, because the goal they have is to live until this day, and to enjoy the celebration one more time. It will literally keep them alive, against the odds, until the goal has been realised.

Our mind naturally works with goals

As you write out your goal, immediately your conscious mind accepts it, while your subconscious mind goes to work to help to turn the goal into a reality. It has been stated in various studies that with goals we have purpose and direction, because our mind is a goal-seeking mechanism, whereas without goals we drift and flounder. The fact that goals give us purpose, direction and energy may explain why all successful people have goals and actively set goals for themselves. Goal-setting is a very important and extremely easy skill that boasts excellent results. Many of us have no idea how important goal-setting is and miss out on its benefits. Rather than dreading ageing, your goals will allow you to plan to age excellently and to stay young and vibrant throughout your life. Your goals will enable you to influence and control the direction of changes that go on as you age, and instead of fearing all the changes and seeing them as unavoidable you will be able to control and postpone many of them.

As you set your goals, remember that what the mind can conceive and believe it can also achieve. Your mind takes everything you say as a command, so make your goals absolutely clear, as described in Step Six. Make sure there is no room whatsoever for misinterpretation. If you instructed a decorator to decorate your house and then left them to it, they would do what they thought you wanted, but would probably misinterpret your desires and give you a result you were not happy with. Think of your mind as a super-efficient assistant; let it know exactly what you want and you are far more likely to get exactly what you want. You must be ready to learn new ways of thinking, behaving, talking and reacting. You must create a goal that is detailed, and you must write it all out clearly.

Step by step towards your goals

There is so much more to goal-setting and achieving than simply writing it out as if it were a wish list on Amazon. Your goal must be a plan, a step-by-step technique in order for it to be realised. Follow these steps to become successful at goal-setting and achieving:

1 SET YOUR GOAL

First set your goal. An example could be, 'I am going to live every day of my life feeling and looking ten years younger.'

2 FORM A CLEAR IMAGE OF IT

Vision is vital to goal-achieving. See it and visualise it clearly, as if it were already in existence. When Mark Victor Hanson wanted his book, *Chicken Soup for the Soul*, to be a best-seller, he cut out the *New York Times* best-seller book list, Tippexed out the number-one entry, and typed *Chicken Soup for the Soul* in its place. Then he stuck it on his bathroom mirror and looked at it every day. By doing this, he was visualising it and, having struggled to get his book published, and then really struggled to make it sell, it went on to be a phenomenal best-seller. The more you visualise, the more you believe, the more it is possible. Really successful people visualise all the time. Vision is vital to goal-achieving – see yourself as phenomenal in the area of delaying ageing so that you excite your imagination and have the drive, determination and sense of certainty that you can and will look and feel younger.

A lovely example of the power of goals was the time when Whoopi Goldberg received an Oscar. She held it up and said to the crowd, 'I have dreamed of this since I was a girl', and then she told the story of how, as an impoverished child she had a goal of being a famous movie star and getting an Oscar, while everyone around her told her she was crazy. She spoke to the audience, and especially to other children who had been like her, and said, 'Never be afraid to have a big vision' – and she was right.

3 COMMIT IT TO PAPER

Write out your goal in detail, so that your subconscious mind has a clear image of what you want and can motivate you to move towards it. Also, write out all the things you are going to do to achieve your goal, from playing your downloaded script from this book (see pages 154–5), to refusing to listen to people who tell you that you cannot slow ageing, to refusing to criticise yourself or use ageing language, to eating healthier food, drinking more water and taking exercise regularly. Plan what you will do to become young, such as adopting the physiology of the young.

4 GET INTO THE HABIT OF LOOKING AT YOUR GOAL EVERY DAY

Place your written goal somewhere you will always see it, and remember that, as you repeat this goal to yourself, your inner resources are already beginning to move towards it. Your goals will change, so update them and rewrite them regularly.

5 WRITE OUT THE REASONS YOU HAVE FOR WANTING TO ACHIEVE THIS GOAL

The more reasons you come up with, the more you will excite your imagination, and the more you will believe it is attainable.

6 SEE YOUR GOALS

Believe in them, and make your mind concentrate on them. Play them back to yourself like a video, as if they were already in existence. Do this just before you go to sleep.

7 FIND A ROLE MODEL

You might want to find a picture of someone who is a great role model for you, an example of ageless ageing, and stick it next to your written goal so that you look at this image daily along with your goal statement. Or find a picture of you at your most active doing some form of activity or sport or looking radiant, and put this next to your goal.

8 BE TENACIOUS

Tenacity, stoicism, persistence and determination are vital. Even your most important goal will not work if you give up too soon, so be persistent. Persistence is a measure of your faith in yourself and in your ability to make it succeed.

Summary – Step Seven

Let's recap on what you have learned in this step.

- You have learned the motivating force of goals on a deep subconscious level, and that your mind is a natural goal-seeking device that will take you towards whatever you focus on, when you focus on it, in a precise, specific and detailed way that brings the desired results.
- You have learned the difference between affirmations and goals:

  - Affirmations are short, precise and to the point; they are often just a sentence or phrase, or a few phrases, designed to be repeated out loud so that they affect the subconscious mind.
  - Goals are something you focus on and move towards by

writing them out, rewriting them as a plan and writing out the plan to accomplish them. You hold the goal in your conscious mind, and make plans to achieve it, while your subconscious mind also accepts the goal and moves you towards it.

It may seem that you have a lot to do, but some of the things you are doing, such as affirmations, become a way of life and are not a form of work at all. Remember:

If you aren't taking action to get younger, you are getting older.

Choose a Script for Becoming Younger

'Youth is a circumstance you can't do anything about.
The trick is to grow up without getting old'

Frank Lloyd Wright (1867–1959)

In this step we are going to go over some varied scripts, each one dealing with a particular aspect of ageing. By now you will be getting used to your own personal programme that you have created. The difference between your programme and these scripts is that your programme is something created just for you. It should be short, just a few paragraphs, and easy to memorise, so that you can think about it and repeat it to yourself regularly at any time.

The scripts are longer and more detailed and have been designed for everyone, but they are also specific to you, they contain biological information and terms, and they are spoken in the third person purposefully. It may seem that you have a lot to do, but you will soon get used to saying your affirmations out loud or reading them from your mirror or computer screen and looking at your goals a few times a week, while looking at your collage/mood board. The scripts can be listened to prior to sleeping, and once they have become embedded in your mind – which takes about three weeks – you no longer have to listen to them every night, just once a week is enough.

The scripts/hypnosis sessions are free to download – for details see page iv. After you have chosen a script that is relevant to you, begin to listen to it every day so that your mind will lock on to the words. Since you will be communicating directly with your cells and giving your body commands, you need to hear the word 'you'; for example, '*You* are working more effectively', '*You* are making more collagen', '*You* are becoming stronger.' If it feels unfamiliar, that's OK. You will soon get used to it. The most important thing to know is that you are using a highly successful technique of communicating with your body that gets results.

When you are listening to the pre-recorded scripts, play them daily for at least 21 days, and thereafter once or twice a week, to condition your mind to accept these new beliefs and to imprint them into your memory. You need to keep your eyes shut and to take in all the information while in a subconscious rather than a conscious state. We focus much better with our eyes closed. The critical factor within your mind, which screens your thoughts, shuts down while in hypnosis, so it will not come up with doubts or objections to what you are hearing and will be more receptive.

You don't need to have great knowledge of the way your body works

When listening to these scripts, it is important to know that you don't need to be a dermatologist or biochemist with a perfect knowledge of the workings of your body to get results. I do have clients who say to me, 'When I listen to your CD I don't understand some of the terms or phrases. Does that mean that I won't get such good results?' You will get excellent results, because your body understands the terms completely and perfectly, and it will do the work for you – all you need to do is believe it will work, expect it to work and see the results.

Most people, when asked to place their hands on their stomach, will put their hands over their intestines because that's where they think of it as being, although it is actually under the ribs. This inability to place body parts correctly does not stop them working. You don't need a full knowledge of how your body works in order to have it work even better, in fact a knowledge of the mind–body connection in making changes will be more beneficial to you than a biological map of the body.

If your doctor were to say to you, 'You have an inflamed pituitary gland or a problem with your cranium', you may be in the dark in terms of locating those body parts and understanding what his diagnosis means, but your mind, on hearing the diagnosis, can manifest all the symptoms that match the diagnosis, despite the fact that you are not consciously visualising this, because you don't understand the language or medical jargon. In the same way children can hear a parent say, 'I have irritable bowel syndrome/lactose intolerance/diverticulitis', and although children don't understand these words they can still develop similar, or even identical, symptoms because they mirror their parents on a level that is above words. Children often resonate on a level that matches their parents' experiences rather than their words.

Concentrate on one script at a time

From the list of scripts below, choose one that is relevant and appealing to you, and listen to it every day until your mind is absolutely familiar with it. You may find that you are interested in more than one script and that even several are of interest to you. If this is the case, you must still focus on one script for 21 days, then, when you have completed it, move on to another, again for 21 days. Don't interchange scripts, or you will dilute the effect. Just concentrate on one script at a time. Later on, when you are listening to the scripts once or twice a month, or once a week, to keep the material in your mind, you can interchange them. You could also create your own script by taking sections from the scripts below and making one that is relevant to you.

1 Script for a younger, healthier body with vitality and energy.
2 Script for staying mentally young with a superb memory.
3 Script for weight reduction.
4 Script for cell regeneration and younger skin.

Exercise 13: Choose and use a script

You now need to go through each script and choose one that you feel is most relevant to you and then to read it to yourself, before you begin playing it to yourself for 21 days. The script for cell regeneration and younger skin can be found in Step Nine – How to Extend Your Cell-by Date (see page 187).

---

1 SCRIPT FOR A YOUNGER, HEALTHIER BODY WITH VITALITY AND ENERGY

As you relax and absorb these words, your inner mind, the most powerful part of you, is now locking on to them and accepting them easily as you become more and more aware that you have a strong desire, and a powerful motivation and ability, to look and feel healthy, vibrant, energetic and younger – to actually become younger.

▶

You are an example of youthfulness. You express yourself as young; you embody the expression of youthful because you think, act, feel and react as ageless, you feel young and you have a wonderful enthusiasm for life. You are looking forward to your future – there is so much for you to plan for and enjoy. Rather than reminiscing about the good old days, you are excited about life today, tomorrow and in the future.

You love life and you love yourself and this is expressed in your zest and enthusiasm for life. You hold in your mind an image of you enjoying excellent health, in which you are active and agile. You have vigour and vitality, and an abundance of energy that favourably impresses everyone you come into contact with. You are an excellent role model for ageless ageing.

You have a passion for life and you take on new activities without paying any attention to your age. Each day you are moving towards the image of you as energetic, full of vitality, youth and health that you hold in your mind so clearly. You are becoming a walking, talking, breathing example of your image of yourself as young, and you become more so every day. You and your cells are working as a perfect team. As you look after your body, your body looks after you. As you inspire your cells, you feel inspired. Your cells are becoming imprinted with your thoughts. You can feel the life force of your cells in every gland, nerve and tissue of your body. You have a constant feeling of rejuvenation.

You are communicating with the intelligence of your cells and directing each cell to function as a young healthy cell now and always. Every cell in your body is a conscious being. Each of your cells is intelligent

▶

and is responding to your thinking, as you think about becoming younger, fitter, active and agile.

Your ability to think these thoughts, to see these things and to accept these suggestions about your health and agility is having a powerful effect on your cells right now. You are able to stimulate your mind and body into action, knowing you don't need to see it specifically – just thinking of it is causing your inner mind to picture it and manifest it perfectly.

Each cell generation is growing strong and resilient and perfect. Your cells grow younger and healthier because you instruct them to; your cells replace themselves with even more perfect cells. See your cells now as glowing, healthy, youthful, perfect, radiant, resilient cells perfectly tuned to other cells, communicating perfectly so that every cell is in the right place at the right time, working perfectly for you with wonderful results.

As you hear these words, each one is making a deep, lasting impression on your mind and replacing every negative belief with a new, constructive one. My voice is going with you, staying embedded in you, having a permanent, powerful and all-pervasive healing effect on you.

2 SCRIPT FOR STAYING MENTALLY YOUNG WITH A SUPERB MEMORY

As you relax and absorb these words you are aware that you are making changes in your life that allow you to maintain a wonderful, alert mind; you take vitamins,

▶

exercise regularly and think positive thoughts, and you adopt positive beliefs which, in turn, are having an excellent effect on your memory. You are communicating with your brain cells, activating within them an ability and desire to function and perform as perfectly as they did in your youth.

Your memory is becoming better and better. Mentally, you are so sharp and agile; you have a wonderful memory and your recall is impressive. You use your mind, because your mind is rather like a muscle: the more you use it the better it is. You know that your mind can't wither as long as you keep introducing it to new things. Your mind cannot get old. Your actions, combined with your positive and powerful belief system, are causing you to have a wonderful, reliable, dependable memory. Everything you hear or see or experience is recorded in your computer-like mind.

Your mind is as efficient as the smartest computer. Like a computer, your mind retains information for you, it stores and holds this information for you and you have perfect and instant access to it. You can remember anything, your memory is outstanding and you have unshakeable confidence and absolute faith in it. You refuse to say things like 'I have forgotten' or 'I can't remember'. Instead you say 'It will come to me any minute now, because I have such a great memory' and it always does. You are running your mind and influencing your memory in the most effective and perfect way.

When you need to remember something, but should it not spring to mind immediately, you give an instruction to your computer-like mind to locate the information

▶

you need and to relay it to you – and it always does. Just like hitting the search button in Google, your mind locates the wealth of information stored in your memory and returns it to you on request. You have wonderful recall and retention. You retain information, facts, figures and memories in your mind perfectly and recall them rapidly and accurately. You need only to ask your subconscious to seek information for you in the same way you would instruct a computer, and within moments the correct information will flow into your conscious mind and stay there for as long as you need it.

You keep your mind active and agile by practising neurobics, by reading a lot and by doing crossword puzzles and brain teasers, and you get the answers right so easily because you have such a capacity to absorb, retain and recall information. You participate in game shows and quizzes set to test your memory, on the radio, television and in newspapers and magazines. The more you do this the better your memory is.

You read all the time, you love reading, you love exciting your imagination, expanding your mind and using your brain. In Russia they say that a person who no longer reads no longer thinks. They also say a person who does not read is no better than one who cannot read and that readers are leaders.

You read, and because you have such a good memory, you read even more. Your conscious mind is expanding, retaining more and more information, which you can immediately recall. You are able to absorb so much material, things you read, hear or experience are all absorbed into your mind and filed

▶

away in a system that is so perfect it delivers this information back to you on demand. You have wonderful powers of concentration, comprehension, retention and recall, and you use them all fully. Whatever you concentrate on you remember. As you get older, your memory remains wonderful, because you remind yourself daily that everything you see, hear and experience is recorded in your mind for your use. You have a perfect memory and perfect recall, your subconscious mind is a filing system, a computer chip of everything you have ever done and it continues to be so throughout your life. You have total faith and absolute confidence in your memory. Whatever is expected tends to be realised, and you expect, with supreme confidence, that your memory will always be superb and your expectations will be met.

You do the things that allow you to maintain a memory that others envy, by exercising to ensure your brain gets a rich supply of oxygen and that the circulation to your brain is good. You pay attention to your digestion and ensure that you absorb nutrients that have a positive impact on your brain functions. You take *Ginkgo biloba* because it improves micro-circulation and is excellent for brain function.

Your brain is a self-rejuvenating organ – the more you use it the better it is. As you work out your body you also work out your brain, memorising routes, poems, instructions and things that interest and inspire you. You tune in to quizzes on the radio and television, and you find your brain answering each question so easily and quickly that you even impress yourself.

Your excellent memory allows you to get older, yet

▶

you know that you are continually making brain cells and memory cells, and that each cell and every neuron and cell receptor is wired up perfectly, resulting in you having a very vital mind. You are mentally young and super-sharp, whatever your years, and will continue to be so.

Every time you use the process of saying 'It will come to me in a second', it does. Every time you use your technique of imagining your memory working as fast and as accurately as a computer, it does. You radiate confidence in your memory. You exude optimism about your memory.

As you hear these words, every word is making a deep, lasting impression on your mind and replacing every negative belief with a new, constructive one. My voice is going with you, staying embedded in you, having a permanent, powerful and all-pervasive healing effect on you.

3 SCRIPT FOR WEIGHT REDUCTION

As you relax and absorb these words you are aware that you have a strong desire and a compelling ability to become slimmer and leaner. This desire and ability is becoming such a powerful part of you that it overrules any old desire to eat destructively, and it constantly motivates you to act in ways that cause you to become and remain at your ideal weight and to become trimmer, healthier, younger and more attractive. You now want only to eat healthy, fresh food. You exercise and you look and feel younger.

▶

You were born with a perfect body and with a perfect attitude to food. As a baby you were so in tune with your body that you knew when to eat and when to stop eating, and you are able to reactivate and reclaim that ability through the power and direction of your inner mind. You knew that you would always have another day to eat and that food would always be available, so you are able to leave food and to say no to the wrong food with ease.

You are becoming more and more in tune with your body, working together as a perfect team. You respond to your body by eating healthy, nutritious food that allows your cells to work perfectly and repair damage while slowing down ageing, while your body responds by becoming leaner, lighter and healthier.

You are aware that you have a right to be slim, you have a drive and commitment to be slim, and daily you feel motivated and conditioned to eat differently, to feel differently about food. You see food as fuel for your body and cells, and you only want to eat the food that your body can use.

You are freeing yourself forever from destructive, self-defeating eating habits. There is no room in your mind or body, or in your life, for overeating. From now on overeating is something you used to do and it cannot, will not and does not, influence you any longer, as you move on from one great achievement to another, by eating differently, becoming leaner, having more energy, exercising willingly and loving the feeling of fitting into smaller clothes and feeling such a sense of accomplishment and achievement.

You have decided to change your weight, shape and size, and you easily take all the action that makes this

▶

happen. You are erasing, eliminating and eradicating poor eating habits forever, as you find yourself refusing to eat the type and amount of food that can only harm your body.

You love your body, so you want to take care of it, and you always treat it with respect. You choose healthy food and eat less food automatically.

See yourself in your mind at your ideal weight. Feel how slim you are. Hear other people praising you on your achievement. Notice how much happier your body is now that you respect it and like it and want to do things that keep it in a healthy, attractive state.

Make an image of how you want to look, and tell your mind that this is what you want. As you focus on this image every day you are already moving towards it, because your mind is picking up that your strongest desire is to reach and maintain this size, shape and weight.

You are now a selective and moderate eater. Old eating habits are fading away forever, leaving you free to eat in a healthy way; leaving you slimmer, more vital, attractive and youthful. Your mind – the most powerful healing force there is – is releasing from you your old overeating habits. You are moving so far, far away from emotional overeating that you can even feel it and sense it shrinking, disappearing, going . . . gone.

As you eat differently, your body is becoming a more super-efficient fat-burning machine using the healthy calories you take in to build a perfect body for you and nourishing your cells with natural food, lean protein and vegetables.

Your metabolic rate is increasing through the power and direction of your mind. Feel, believe and imagine

▶

your metabolic rate working as perfectly as it did in your childhood.

Your stomach is shrinking. Your stomach is the size of your fist, so begin to squeeze your fist while repeating to yourself over and over again, 'My stomach is the size of my fist. My stomach is the size of my fist.' Notice your stomach shrinking – feel it becoming smaller now. As you concentrate on this feeling it will increase through the power and direction of your mind. Your stomach is becoming small, tiny, and you find yourself eating enough food to satisfy that capacity of a fist and then stopping easily and willingly, because you want to.

From now on you eat only in response to real hunger. You are now and forever a sensible and selective eater. You drink a lot of water every day to assist your body in eliminating excess weight. You crave water and drink eight glasses a day. Your skin is glowing. You feel fabulous.

You leave some food at every meal, because you feel full quite quickly. You eat slowly and you love that feeling of choice. You always leave something. It makes you feel powerful and healthy. Food cannot control you because you are taking charge of how you eat, how you look and how you feel. You have a positive attitude to your body and an overwhelming ability to become slim.

You understand that if your body needed excess food it wouldn't turn it into excess body weight. Excess food is wasted wherever it goes. You refuse to treat your body as a rubbish bin, and you leave excess food or throw it away with glee. You know that overeating is punishing to your body. Your body and cells hate being overworked with too much food.

▶

You know that sugar is your enemy: it ages your skin and makes your body store fat, so you become indifferent to sugar. It thrills you, delights you and elates you to say no to sugar, and you do this all the time. You effortlessly and continuously say no to sugar and yes to looking and feeling young. You choose to do this, and you choose to feel great about it too.

You love your body. Your body loves you back and is becoming more and more the way you want it to be. As you do this wonderful thing for your body – saying no to sugar and yes to eating selectively – your body does so many wonderful things for you and you look and feel amazing. Every day you are nourished, filled and satisfied by the good feelings you have about yourself, and your appetite is changing in the most perfect way. You need less nourishment from food because you are emotionally nourished. You eat less, but you enjoy the food you eat more. You eat slowly, you eat less and you always choose lean, nutritious and healthy food that your body easily digests.

As you eat in this healthy, wonderful way, your body uses every perfect calorie to rebuild and rejuvenate you, and you become leaner, slimmer and radiantly healthy. You look younger and fitter. Your clothes look so much better on you. Because you feel so good about yourself, you exercise and treat your body with love and respect. You easily reach a body weight that is right and appropriate for you. Eating healthy food and exercising is becoming a fundamental, integral part of you. It is another way of you being good to yourself, reclaiming a positive self-image and loving yourself.

It is natural for you to eat healthy food, because you

▶

are using your power of choice to choose how you are going to feel and look. You have chosen to eat differently and to become slimmer easily and permanently. Now, visualise an image of this, then see and feel your stomach as smaller and flatter, your thighs as leaner, your waist as smaller, because you have made up your mind and set your mind to reach and maintain your ideal weight.

Each of these words makes a deep, vivid and permanent impression on your subconscious. Every day you become more aware of the full, powerful effect these words are having on you. The healing power of your own mind is strengthening and perfecting your ability to change your weight and eating habits. As you absorb these words you are reinforcing your mind, replacing every negative belief with a new, constructive one. My voice is going with you, staying embedded in you, having a permanent, powerful and all-pervasive, healing effect on you.

In order to score your success at taking control of how you age, and chart your progress, I want you to test yourself using the quiz below. You will find that when you repeat the test after using the philosophy in this book that you get a much better score. You will also become aware, as you go through each question, of the changes you can make that will give you a better score and a younger body and mind.

Test for ageing successfully

Give yourself one point for each statement to which you can respond 'yes'. Add up your score and read your assessment at the end of the test.

1   I am happy most of the time.
2   I like my body and feel a sense of health and well-being in it.
3   I have a passion for life.
4   I feel young.
5   I am involved in young activities (sport, games, dancing, and so on).
6   I am able to have fun and enjoy doing things without needing to pay any attention to my age.
7   I am able to choose my thoughts and language and to influence how I feel.
8   My identity is completely separate from my age.
9   I do new things and look forward to my future while living in the moment.
10 I change my beliefs to suit my life. I let go of beliefs that are outdated, fixed or rigid.
11 I am flexible in my attitude and opinions.
12 I exercise for at least 30 minutes, three times a week and I generally enjoy it.
13 I feel energetic after eating.
14 I am within 10 per cent of my ideal weight.
15 I eat fresh food, drink lots of water and take vitamins and supplements (see page 229). I eat less sugar and starchy carbohydrates, more protein and vegetables.
16 I don't overeat and I don't eat late at night very often.
17 My digestion is good.
18 My diet contains lots of vegetables and oily fish.
19 I am able to limit the amount of alcohol I drink.
20 I consume less than three cups of coffee a day.
21 I skin brush and exfoliate regularly (see page 259).
22 I always use a sunscreen and avoid the direct sun.
23 I don't smoke.
24 I don't have any major fears in my life.
25 I breathe properly and enjoy taking deep breaths.
26 Fear of ageing is not something I focus on any longer.

27   I don't use drugs (stimulants, tranquillisers, antidepressants).
28   I have a happy family life.
29   I get along with people at work and out of work.
30   I enjoy friendships.
31   I sleep easily at night for more than six hours without needing pills or alcohol.
32   I wake up feeling refreshed after restful sleep.
33   I sleep with just one fairly flat pillow (see page 263).
34   I get to sleep before midnight most nights and before 2.00 a.m. even more frequently.
35   I restrict electrical appliances in my bedroom and especially around my bed (see page 243).
36   I feel good about my physical well-being.
37   I feel good about my emotional and psychological well-being.
38   I feel good about my financial well-being.
39   Minor challenges, such as traffic jams, being late, missing an appointment, and so on, are things I take in my stride.
40   I usually see the positive side of things.
41   I find something to laugh about daily.
42   I am able to laugh at myself.
43   I am not often in a hurry.
44   I can usually control my time rather than it controlling me.
45   I am mentally active. I enjoy reading, writing, keeping up with current affairs, and so on.
46   I am flexible and can adjust to changes quite easily.
47   I am not rigid in my thoughts about how things must be. I am open to change; I willingly update my thoughts and beliefs.
48   I can commit myself to a task, job or project.
49   I can commit myself to a relationship.
50   I love my job.
51   I have moments of feeling so happy and carefree.
52   I am able to enjoy silence and calmness on a daily basis,

meditating, using self-hypnosis, yoga or periods of reflection and quiet.

53 I feel very loved.
54 I have a good sex life.

Award yourself one point for every statement to which you responded with 'yes'.

Score:
Over 45: exceptional.
35–45: excellent.
25–34: good, but pay attention to missing factors to age well.
Under 25: rethink and restructure your priorities by taking action in the areas you answered with 'no'.

Take this test again a few weeks after you have made the lifestyle changes, and you will find that you get a higher score.

I hope you have enjoyed listening to these scripts. The script for cell regeneration therapy and younger skin can be found in Step Nine. I want you to listen to one every day and you will soon see the results.

Summary – Step Eight

Let's recap what you have learned in this step.

- You have learned the power of scripts and how something written and put together in a particular format can have an immediate as well as progressive effect on the mind and body. You have learned more about how to excite and activate your imagination.
- You have taken a test that will show you how you are ageing and, by now, you will have some very real and definite

changes going on in your body, both externally and internally.

- You can feel proud of yourself for staying with the programme and taking each step. As you begin to see and feel results you will know it is worth it, not just for now but for 10, 20 and 30 years from now, when you will still be benefiting from them.

'If you were to destroy in mankind the belief in immortality not only love but every living force maintaining the life of the world would at once be dried up'

Fyodor Dostoevsky (1821–81)

How to Extend Your Cell-by Date

'An inordinate passion for pleasure is the secret of
remaining young'

Oscar Wilde (1854–1900)

Ageing begins to happen when our system breaks down through
free-radical damage. Free radicals are rogue cells that contain
oxygen in an active form. Oxidation is the combination of oxygen
and molecules; unstable molecules are free radicals and are
needed to destroy bacteria, parasites and virus-infected cells, but
they also damage healthy cells and cause them to malfunction and
degenerate. This oxygen-based damage to cells is a major factor in
ageing, but it can be counteracted by taking antioxidants and
eating foods that are rich in free-radical scavengers and by visualising free-radical scavengers surging through the body depleting
free radicals. In the same way that oxidation will rust a car or
turn food mouldy, it will age our bodies, but we can do a great
deal to slow this down.

Scientists in Kentucky and Oklahoma injected older gerbils
with a chemical compound that neutralised the effects of oxygen-
based damage to cells and found the gerbils began to grow
younger. Even their memory reversed to that of younger gerbils.

In Dallas, similar tests have been carried out on fruit flies, and the findings have shown that when the fruit fly's cells are protected against oxygen-based damage, their lifespan increases by a third.

Scientists at the Biology of Aging Program at The National Institute on Aging in Maryland, USA, believe we could live to 120 years if we could prevent the molecular damage happening in our cells. If our cells repaired and replaced themselves perfectly each time, every cell would be perfect and new, and we would never grow old. Cells have to divide to multiply, and each new cell is encoded with all the information it needs to function perfectly. The number of times a cell replaces itself is very important to ageing. Eventually, cells stop reproducing. If they did not do this, we would actually never age.

By using cell regeneration you can speed up the process and keep your cells in a better, younger condition, as well as considerably slowing down and delaying the time when cells cease to work to their optimum.

What happens as cells degenerate?

Ageing also begins to occur when cells cease to function at peak efficiency, which in turn leads to a breakdown in cell communication. Once cells stop communicating at peak efficiency all kinds of damage occurs in the body. We die because our bodies contain so many specialised cells that they can no longer undergo the rejuvenating influence of cell division. Death is the result of wear and tear within un-dividing cells that can no longer repair the damage.

Cells are constantly renewing and replacing themselves at a rate of millions every second. However, most human cells can only copy themselves 50 to 60 times before they die. The reason for programmed cell death lies in our chromosomes, the 46 strands of DNA found at the heart of almost every cell. The ends of every chromosome are protected by a chemical cap called a telomere. They act like the plastic tips on the end of shoelaces and stop the strands of DNA from fraying. However, each time a human cell divides, these telomeres get shorter. Eventually – after 50 or so divisions – they are too short to protect the chromosomes and the cell dies.

Telomeres shorten as we age but a pilot study, published in *The Lancet Oncology,* found that the telomeres of people who switch to a healthier lifestyle – by making changes to diet, reducing stress and undertaking moderate exercise – can be lengthened by an average of 10 per cent, effectively reversing the natural ageing process.[6]

The study's leader, Professor Dean Ornish, from the Preventive Medicine Research Institute at the University of California in San Francisco, said: 'If validated by large-scale randomised controlled trials, these comprehensive lifestyle changes may significantly reduce the risk of a wide variety of diseases and premature mortality. Our genes, and our telomeres, are a predisposition, but they are not necessarily our fate.'

Dr Lynne Cox of the University of Oxford said: 'This new study suggests that reducing stress, improving diet and increasing exercise not only prevent telomere loss but also lead to small but significant increases in telomere length.'

More studies show that your lifestyle can influence by two-thirds the rate at which your telomeres shorten. Stressors, such as eating unhealthy food, smoking, drinking and lack of exercise, increase cell damage and can chip away at telomeres. A 2012 study in the journal *PLoS One* found that middle-aged and older women who suffered with acute anxiety had shorter telomeres than women who weren't anxious.[7]

The same healthy behaviours that are good for your heart can increase levels of telomerase, an enzyme in the body that can rebuild some of your telomeres. A study published in the journal *Psychoneuroendocrinology* reported that people who meditated boosted their telomerase levels significantly.[8] In another study,

Ohio State University researchers found that overweight, sedentary adults who took supplements containing either 2.5g or 1.25g of active omega-3 polyunsaturated fatty acids daily for four months actually lengthened their telomeres. Lowering stress levels by listening to the scripts in this book can lengthen your life by stalling telomere decline.

In essence, our cells are like miniature factories processing nourishment and voiding waste, and the quality of our health relates directly to the quality of the health of our cells. Our cells are constantly replacing themselves, but because of this breakdown in communication, a damaged cell will replace itself with a damaged cell, despite the fact that it has the blueprint – the DNA – to replace itself with a perfect cell.

The mind can regenerate our cells

We can reactivate this communication by talking to our cells. It almost sounds too simple, I know, but, as I have explained earlier, our cells hear every word we say and already react to these words. Therefore, if you were to use a programme where you spoke to your cells in a particular format designed to make your cells work better and to continue to communicate with each other, you would be able to prevent much of the breakdown of cell communication and the damage that results from it while keeping your cells working at peak efficiency for longer.

Since our cells respond to our thinking, and respond extremely well to direct mental commands, it is possible to communicate with cells, to talk to them. We already know that our cells hear and respond to our thoughts. Cell regeneration therapy will enable you to communicate with your cells in a much more direct way. You will be able to tell your cells what to do, to command them to work as they are designed to work and to have them act accordingly. This programme will allow you to command and instruct your cells to return to their original blueprint and coding, and to function perfectly and properly as they were intended to do.

The mind is able to trigger cell communicators, thus allowing cells to communicate more effectively with each other and, as a result of this, to function more efficiently. Even our immune system responds to our thinking and to our beliefs. It also responds to the way we see our ability to take control of events and will respond as you take control of how you plan to age.

Each cell is capable of replacing itself with a perfect cell for longer, and this can considerably delay the onset of ageing. As you listen to the script on cellular regeneration in this chapter you will be able to communicate with your cells. You can memorise it by reading it frequently and by playing the download.

PERFECT CELLS CAN REPLACE DAMAGED CELLS

Every one of your trillions of cells is perfectly able to repair and rejuvenate itself, and also to replace itself with a perfect cell. Damaged cells can be programmed to replace themselves with perfect cells, because our cells are intelligent and, in addition, they are directed by an inner intelligence. Within each cell is the electrical coding that imprints the function and purpose of that cell and is the blueprint for perfect cell replacement. Because of the cell's particular intelligence, it requires only a form of communication with the cell's intelligence, a direction, instruction or command, to activate the cell's ability to repair or replace itself perfectly.

Our emotions have the power to create illness or good health

The mind is stronger than medicine, because our muscles, nerves and cells hear and respond to every word we say. Our emotions affect the blood flow and the endocrine system. We can direct our healing intelligence to free, to move, to shrink, to reduce and to minimise ailments and the signs of ageing.

Cells have an innate intelligence of their own and make decisions below the level of our awareness. Despite the fact that we are not consciously aware of these decisions, we nevertheless still have a vast ability to influence them.

Norman Cousins (1915–90) called placebos 'the doctor that resides within you'. There is a pharmacist within each of us that can make the chemicals you need to stay younger, and as you communicate with this 'inner pharmacist' through your cells you will slow down ageing.

The mind manifests itself through the body, and feelings of joy are transferred from organ to organ, as are feelings of worry, pain or unhappiness. Worry can transform itself into ulcers, throat problems, stomach pains, poor skin and a host of other ailments. Anxiety transfers itself from organ to organ in the body. The body is very aware of anxiety and cells hold on to the memory of anxiety and then remind you of it through feelings, even when you think you have consciously forgotten it. Feelings of anger stimulate the adrenal glands and the increased adrenaline in the blood causes many changes in the body.

Neuropeptides, which are chemical messengers, travel through the body every time we think a thought or speak a word. Negative thoughts create poisonous neuropeptides; where a thought goes a chemical goes with it, and where a thought goes energy flows.

Neuropeptides and transmitters link up to our thoughts, and all our thoughts turn into molecules. These molecules make decisions within the body that relate to our thoughts, although no one yet knows exactly how this works. When we are rushed, tense and anxious, we speed up ageing and become biologically older, whereas when we are calm we slow it down.

HATE OR LOVE – EMOTIONS THAT DIRECTLY INFLUENCE OUR HEALTH

If you do something but hate it, you will make chemicals that weaken your immune system. If you continuously do something you hate, your body will pay a high price for this. It will suffer because you hate what you are doing. If you regularly and consistently do things that you hate, you will begin to hate your life.

If you do the same thing and love it, on the other hand, you will make very different chemicals, and these will boost your immune system.

We can't always learn to love the things we hate, but we can learn to attach less powerful feelings to them. It's important to accept something and look for some positive aspects of it or to change it. The worse thing we can do is to get into the vicious circle of 'I can't accept it and I can't change it', or 'I hate this but I have got to do it'.

Believing and saying 'I can't accept this and I am unable to do anything about it' will make you feel powerless. That feeling can, in turn, cause your body to *feel* powerless and to act or behave in a powerless way.

If you feel like this about anything at all – be it your job, how you look, or even doing the ironing – I recommend you either change how you feel about it and look for some positive aspects of it, and then decide to feel better about it, or change something about it. Whatever you decide to do, just knowing that you can choose to attach different feelings and language to anything at all will help you.

When I was driving my daughter to school some years ago, the bridge I drove over daily was reduced from three lanes to one for almost a year, making the journey take three times as long and involving a lot of stationary traffic. After several months of this slow, time-consuming crawl I noticed I was saying, 'This is annoying, frustrating and stressful' to myself on a daily basis – I was beginning to hate the journey, but I had to make a return journey on that route twice every day.

Then one day I stopped myself, noticed how I was thinking, and decided that I must change this, which I did, by reminding myself that I had chosen this school and chosen to drive my daughter there every day, because it was important to her. I couldn't change the drive to school, so instead I had to change how I felt about it.

I looked at people waiting for the bus and remembered I was lucky to have a car. I don't enjoy being stuck in traffic, but I no longer called it stressful, it's just traffic, and I made a point of using that time, which I had been thinking of as a waste of time, to listen to CDs or have conversations with my daughter or just to think. I even bought myself one of those plastic cup holders that sticks between the seats and made myself some tea, which I could enjoy in the car each morning as the traffic crawled along, and something as simple as that made a big difference.

OUR INTERPRETATION OF EVENTS IS WHAT CAUSES STRESS TO THE BODY

We all say things like 'It's so stressful raising children/commuting to work/dealing with colleagues/dealing with the boss/relatives' – the list is endless – and although everything we are saying might be true, it is important to attach less stress to it and to use different words.

The way we define and interpret events affects our cell receptors. It's never what has actually happened that counts but the meaning we attach to it. A negative view of things raises our cortisol levels and causes us to feel more pain.

As I have said before, it's important to attach a different meaning to ageing and to see every stage as challenging and exciting. Consciously attach a different meaning to events that you have perceived as stressful; if you cannot change the event, you must change the meaning you attach to it, and by doing something as simple as this you can change your life. Even when you feel there is nothing you can change, you *can* change your thoughts.

Remember too that what you are seeing as stressful may be someone else's dream come true. They might love to have a stressful experience of being under too much pressure at work, or to own a car so that they could experience the traffic, or just to have a family.

A Croatian girl stayed with me during the Bosnian crisis. She came with me to my local supermarket and started to cry. She was sending food parcels back to her family, because they had nothing. She wanted to spend hours looking at all the variety of food and kept saying, 'You are so lucky, you have so much choice, so much food, you must love coming here. If I was you I would like to come here every day.' She attached a very different meaning to being in this shop than did most of the other shoppers, who were looking harassed and keen to get in and out as quickly as they could.

Deepak Chopra describes going on a rollercoaster ride at a funfair: one person might hate it and find it scary. They would be making cortisol and adrenaline, which can destroy the immune system. Another would go on that same ride, love it, find it thrilling and exhilarating and would be making interleukin 2, which is a most powerful anti-cancer drug.

A very famous rock star was describing what it was like to perform on stage and said, 'Before I go on stage my heart starts to beat really fast, my palms sweat, adrenaline pumps through me and I feel so excited I can't wait to go out there and perform.' Compare this with another famous performer who gave up performing live after describing this: 'When I was about to go on stage awful things started happening to my body, I would get a rapid heartbeat, adrenaline would rush through me, I would feel sweaty and nervous and I realised I was having panic attacks. Eventually I had to give up live performances because the panic attacks would not go away, and then I gave up singing altogether.'

The feelings and sensations of each performer are so similar, but the interpretation is completely different, and the chemicals each performer's body manufactured would be different largely because of these opposite interpretations.

Information is passed from one cell to the next generation

If you use ageing language, if your identity of yourself is old or ageing, then your DNA will pass on through each cell generation the belief that you are old or ageing. The same is true with weight and addictions. If your language and thoughts are all along the lines of 'I can't lose weight. I can't eat like other people do' then you are passing on that information from one cell to the next.

Cells remember addictions, weight patterns and anxieties, and this information is passed on through each new cell generation. The memory of the addiction or the excess weight can therefore persist in new cells even years later. By using cell regeneration therapy you can change this forever.

INFLUENCE YOUR CELLS WITH ONLY GOOD BELIEFS

The worst beliefs are the kind that tell us that 'Other people can do that, but I can't', or 'Other people can look younger, but I can't.' You can, and this programme will make sure of that, but you also must believe that you can, so that your cells are able to believe that you can.

Your cells are not able to disagree with you and they accept everything you say and even think as a fact, so you have nothing to lose and everything to gain by telling yourself and your cells the opposite. Tell yourself you look and feel ageless every day and you will become ageless. I can hear you again saying, 'This sounds too easy. If it's so easy, why isn't everyone doing it?' It's a good question, but more and more people are understanding the power of thought and using it to make wonderful changes in their lives.

Our bodies are run by a labyrinth, an organisation of intelligence with information continuously being sent out and received, and by using relaxation methods, the power of thought and visualisation techniques we can go deep enough to positively influence this organisation of intelligence, and to change body patterns and influence cells so that we can enjoy better health and longevity. Just listening to the downloads provided with this book will do this for you.

How my cell regeneration therapy evolved

In my practice as a hypnotherapist, for years I have been going on a journey into the body with my patients and communicating with their cells, then activating the body's ability to heal and repair itself. Some of the results have been outstanding, especially with patients who have had chronic illnesses.

I began to study the effects this technique – which I called 'cell regeneration therapy' – had on ageing, and they were equally impressive. I travelled across the US studying with experts in the ageing process and gathering information for this book.

In the West we have been taught to hand over our bodies and our ailments to the medical profession, and we give them the responsibility for making us well, and yet we have more power to heal, to fix and to change our bodies than any outside source. Doctors can do wonderful work, especially in the area of surgery, but in the area of healing the body you can make the healing chemicals needed, you only need to be shown how to do it. Your body can heal and repair itself in many areas and it can slow down and arrest ageing.

A case has been documented of a teenager who lost her heel in a motorbike accident and, using a form of hypnosis, commanded her body to grow a new left heel, using the right heel as a model – and she did, successfully, regrow her heel.

Healthy tissue has been regrown and burns healed without scarring, using the same process. What you think is possible affects your body.

Deepak Chopra says, 'We can interrupt the past pattern of ageing at a cellular level, then the DNA can work its miracles, our intelligence is so willing to provide this.'[9]

Exercise 14: Regenerate your cells

1   Practise using your mind to trigger cell communication so that your cells are strong and communicate perfectly with each other. Read the script on cell regeneration therapy on page 187, then close your eyes and visualise all your cells in the right place at the right time, doing their perfect work.

2   Communicate with your cells to activate their ability to repair, renew and replace themselves at peak efficiency. Talk to your cells and tell them what you want and expect from them. Tell your cells to behave in a way that will allow you to stay young.

The more you do this, the more you will be using your mind to trigger cell communicators so that your cells work more efficiently. Remember that a form of interplay or communication is always going on between your mind and body, so what you are doing is not so unusual – it's not even new. You already engage in a form of self-communication quite unconsciously, and now you are ready to do it consciously and to love the benefits.

▶

You can talk to your cells the way you might talk to a very bright ten-year-old child, giving them clear and easy-to-follow instructions, telling them how you want them to behave. Using this programme you will tell your cells to act as young healthy cells in a more direct, beneficial and positive way. The key is to use the points below as you communicate with your cells and any other part of you:

a   Talk to your cells in the present tense, and use only positive words. Say 'grow younger and healthier, replace yourself with even more perfect cells', rather than saying 'Don't be old or sick.'

b   Be absolutely clear. Show your cells with words and images exactly how you want them to be.

c   Use very descriptive words, such as 'glowing', 'healthy', 'youthful', 'perfect', 'radiant', 'resilient cells perfectly tuned to other cells, communicating perfectly', so that every cell is in the right place at the right time working perfectly with perfect results.

d   Use the present tense as you talk to your cells. Say, 'My cells are becoming stronger. Each cell generation is strong, resilient and perfect.'

e   Be as detailed as you can. Imagine your cells and metabolic rate acting as efficiently as they did when you were a child. Imagine that your digestion is perfect. Tell your cells to do the work; tell them how much it means to you and thank them.

f   Communicate with your cells frequently. It is better to spend five minutes communicating with them every day than one hour every ten days.

How I have used self-healing techniques

I was stretching in the gym one evening and I pulled a muscle in my leg so badly that I could hardly walk. I was due to take part in the filming of a television show the very next day, so it was hugely inconvenient and I was worried they would replace me if I could not deliver. Immediately, I began to tell my muscle to heal itself, to rapidly repair itself and to use the other leg as a model to repair itself. I kept visualising my leg as completely healthy and normal and imagining the injured leg muscle looking exactly like the muscle in the other leg, which was perfect. I have no idea what either muscle really looked like, but I knew that was not really important. It did not work immediately, and I was in some pain all evening, but I did not lose faith, I kept on imagining my muscle healing and telling it to heal itself.

A lot of people who learn these healing techniques abandon them because they don't get results immediately and they don't believe they are working. Sometimes it takes longer. There is something called 'lag time', which is the time between you giving the instructions, your body getting the message and the work being completed. Anyway, the next day my leg felt a lot better, but I was still in some discomfort, but the day after that it felt so normal that I had forgotten that I had even pulled a muscle – and then suddenly I remembered and thought, 'Wow this is working – my leg feels absolutely fine!' Even though I have been doing this work for years I still get such a thrill when I use my mind to heal my body, and then notice the results.

Command your body to repair itself

If you wish, you can make your own programme for cell regeneration by referring to everything you have learned about how to programme your mind, and applying these same rules to programming your cells. As I mentioned earlier, your cells are like smart children. They know exactly what to do to allow you to remain young, and they know exactly how to do it, but they have to be commanded, instructed and told what to do in a specific way that causes them to respond to you. Some of my clients really dislike the word 'command', but commanding your body cells to work more productively is the same as instructing them. You can simply talk to your cells the way you might talk to a clever ten-year-old, as we saw above in the previous exercise.

You will see below how to bring about the repair of body tissues as a result of direct mental commands. Note: please don't worry about the length of this script, you don't need to memorise it as you will be playing it to yourself frequently via the download.

---

4 SCRIPT FOR CELL REGENERATION AND YOUNGER SKIN

As you relax your inner mind, the most powerful part of you is now locking on to these words and accepting them easily. You are becoming more and more aware that you have a strong desire and a powerful motivation and ability to look and feel younger, to become younger and to have younger skin and a younger, healthy complexion. You are ready and able to motivate your skin cells to act as younger cells do. You have the power to influence your cells, to communicate with any part of your body, and to have that part respond to your instructions.

You are now using the power of your mind to direct and command your skin cells to act as younger cells do. Because your body is controlled by a network of intelligence, which is influenced by your mind, you are able to relax deeply enough to influence your own

▶

mind and to change patterns of the body and to slow down the ageing process.

You are able to accept only positive ideas about your cells and to imprint this onto your cells.

You are communicating with the intelligence of your cells, directing each cell to function as a young, healthy cell now and always.

Every cell in your body is a conscious being. Each of your cells is intelligent and responds to your thinking, as you think about becoming younger and know that you can look and feel years younger, now and always.

Imagine and know that you can influence cell renewal so that it speeds up and becomes more efficient. As a result of this, ageing slows down. Your ability and willingness to talk to your cells is slowing down ageing right now.

When you were younger, your cells repaired and renewed themselves at peak efficiency. You had perfect cells and your cells have a perfect memory of this. You are able to activate this memory and to set off changes in your cells just by thinking of it. Think of your cells becoming younger now, imagine your cells doing their perfect work at peak efficiency. Imagine and feel your cells performing more effectively so that your skin functions as a younger skin does and will continue to do so. Every time you think these thoughts, each cell is renewing itself with a younger, healthier and stronger cell.

As you relax and think these thoughts, and hear these words, you are able to drift into a different state of consciousness, a state where you are able to penetrate the cell wall to communicate with your DNA – the blueprint for healthy cells.

You are responding wonderfully to direct mental

▶

commands, and enabling each cell to replace itself with a younger, healthier cell, activating the rejuvenating process, by communicating with your cells and increasing cell renewal and regeneration.

Your thoughts are commanding your skin to perform at peak efficiency, as it did in your youth.

Because whatever you focus on you move towards, you are focusing on your connective tissue as supportive, and you are imagining oxygen-rich blood being sent by your subconscious mind to your skin, to feed and nourish it, to feed cells and increase cell renewal even more.

You know that your beliefs create biology, that your thoughts are so powerful that they are creating physical effects within your body right now. You are activating healthy cells through the power of your thinking.

As you relax and take in these words, know that your mind responds to your thinking, to the words and images you make. See your skin as resilient, more supple and elastic, and able to heal and repair itself quickly. Sebum is increasing, your epidermis is remaining thick and your sebaceous glands are staying active, your connective tissue is strong and your skin's immune-response cells work perfectly. Your healing white blood cells are working as perfectly as they did in your childhood.

Your skin cells are regaining and retaining their ability to communicate perfectly with each other, so each cell is able to do its work perfectly, your cell production is increased, surface cells are shedding more quickly, new cells are rapidly coming to the surface, and with this rapid turnover of skin cells your skin looks and feels younger, moist, glossy and healthier.

▶

By frequently focusing on this, you are activating your skin cells and speeding up cell renewal so that your skin has lustre, glow and a smoother, younger appearance. Through cellular communication you are speeding up production of collagen and elastin and encouraging your skin's natural repair process.

Now imagine the surface dead skin cells shedding, see them falling away as dead, dry flakes – as dust. As this happens, new healthy, glossy cells are constantly moving up from the dermis, like perfectly organised ranks, to the skin's surface. You are constantly producing healthy, glowing cells. Your skin looks moist, supple, younger and more healthy, your complexion is clear and glossy.

In younger skin, surface cells are shed every 28 days, so imagine, instruct and command your cells to shed every 28 days, revealing new healthy, younger skin. The dull, dead cells are falling away. Imagine the protein bonds that held the dead cells on the surface, like glue, responding perfectly to your thoughts and freeing up to discard the old cells.

When you exfoliate, you see improved results, your moisturiser works better at protecting your consistent supply of healthy, glossy, plump, moist, firm and young cells. Your skin quality is smoother, firmer and more youthful. Your body cells act as younger cells. Your supportive network of collagen and elastin fibres is strong and will remain so. Even thinking about their strength can increase it, so see your network of collagen and elastin becoming stronger, leaving your skin supple with a smooth surface. Through your imagination and through your creative thinking you are directing your sebum production, ensuring that it is speedy and constant.

▶

As a result, your skin looks and feels moister. Your sebaceous glands stay active to keep your skin moist, and you are able to encourage this by visualising it.

Now think, see and believe in your mind's ability to increase circulation and cell respiration, so that even now your cells are repairing themselves, communicating productively and producing plenty of collagen to help your skin's support system. You help your skin even more by constantly removing negative thoughts and language about ageing from your thinking and your mind.

Your mind is influencing your body, and you are influencing your mind in the most perfect way. You are developing a clear mental image, visualising your skin and skin cells as young and healthy, and knowing that the more you imagine it the more rapidly it will occur. Your ability to think these thoughts, to see these things and to accept these suggestions about your skin, is having a powerful effect on your cells right now. You are able to stimulate your mind and body into action. Remember: you don't need to see it specifically, just thinking of it is causing your inner mind to picture it and manifest it perfectly.

Because your imagination has no limits, you can see and feel your skin as younger, your muscles as tighter and firmer, and any lines as finer. As you do this, you are reinforcing your subconscious mind, replacing negative thoughts with new positive ones. As you focus on achieving younger skin with confidence in your ability to make it happen, you can and will achieve it.

This image of you with younger, firmer skin is becoming more real, more attainable and more clear

▶

each time you hear this script. Your inner mind – the most powerful part of you – is locking on to these words, hearing them over and over again. They are becoming a powerful part of your memory.

Your skin has a natural ability to renew itself – and is doing so every second. You make a new epidermis every month, so see your epidermis replacing itself with a new, thicker epidermis, full of healthy cells ready to do their work perfectly, enabling your skin to retain optimum elasticity.

Now see your skin healing and replenishing itself easily while you make more epidermal skin cells nourished with nutrient-laden blood. Your blood capillaries are strong and healthy, aiding blood flow to the skin.

You are stimulating your circulation and maximising production of new cells by breathing properly and deeply. As you breathe deeply you are increasing the amount of oxygen available to your cells and the elimination of toxins. You are also strengthening your cells and rejuvenating your body while increasing your skin's cycle of cell reproduction so that plump, light-reflecting cells come to the surface more frequently.

The bonds that hold dead cells on the skin's surface are broken easily, revealing a fresh skin that looks hydrated and healthy. Your skin is continually behaving as a young skin does, making collagen and elastin, staying smooth, supple, elastic and firm. Your facial muscles stay strong and work well, supporting your skin.

Every cell in your body is now more perfect, more youthful and more alive. Each cell is replacing itself with a purer, finer, more perfect cell. Dead skin flakes fall away, encouraging new layers of skin cells to form and show as rapidly as they do in younger skin.

▶

Your skin is looking fresher and newer – proof that it is renewing itself at a faster, younger rate. Your complexion is smooth, glossy, youthful and luminous. As you successfully use the power of your mind for cellular regeneration, cell communicators are triggered, leaving your skin moist and satiny with improved skin tone.

Visualise free-radical scavengers working perfectly and effectively to destroy free radicals. See these free-radical scroungers mopping up free radicals and minimising any free-radical damage so that your skin cells are strong and resilient, and they communicate and work perfectly with each other, giving out and receiving the right information.

Your trillions of cells are all in the right place, at the right time, doing the right job, boosting cell renewal, protecting the cell membrane, promoting healthy cell division and activating DNA – and a wonderful skin quality is the result.

You have perfect cell protein, collagen and elastin. Your skin is supported and strong. Now see your muscles as strong, your facial muscles are attached to your skin. See your muscles as taut and your skin as firm. You have excellent circulation and good skin tone and colour, excellent blood and lymph flow, and cells that are rich in oxygen and nutrients. Your muscles act as a support system for your skin. See your muscles as supple and firm as they were in your youth. On top of your muscles, see healthy connective tissue; above this is the dermis and epidermis, which is thick and healthy because it is full of growing cells.

Your skin is firm and supported, new collagen is always forming, every cell is surrounded by connective tissue,

▶

and you see this as elastic, supple and firm with a healthy blood supply keeping your muscles young and elastic.

Because you care about your skin you have a strong desire to keep it in excellent condition. You eat a healthy diet rich in vitamins and antioxidants that guard against cell destruction. You drink eight glasses of water daily, because it is vital for healthy skin. You breathe properly and you use sun block and the best skincare routine for you.

Each night, your cells renew and repair themselves as you sleep, so you feel this and imagine this taking place. As you fall asleep, you focus on and dream of your healthy cells renewing and repairing and benefiting your skin.

As you sleep, your subconscious mind is increasing blood flow to your skin, affecting your skin and skin cells, and affecting you in the most perfect way. You are producing healthy hormones, enabling your skin to function as a young, healthy skin and your cells are becoming super-efficient.

These words are influencing your cells and influencing you in the most positive and safe way, allowing you to achieve younger-looking and younger-functioning skin.

Each of these words makes a deep, vivid and permanent impression on your subconscious. Every day you become more aware of the full, powerful effect these words are having on you. The healing power of your own mind is strengthening and perfecting your ability to influence how you age in a positive way. As you absorb these words you are reinforcing your mind, replacing every negative belief with a new constructive one. My voice is going with you, staying embedded in you, having a permanent, powerful and all-pervasive healing effect on you.

Reclaim and redefine your image of yourself

In this step we are covering one of my favourite subjects: how you can feel great about yourself and how you can literally reclaim and redefine a positive image of yourself. You probably understand by now how powerful the relationship is between your thoughts and your cells and how you can use that to your advantage, by conditioning your cells to continually act as young, healthy cells. One of the best ways to have healthy cells is to have a healthy attitude to yourself and to truly love your body. It is not good enough to love only a part of your body – the parts that you like and accept or feel are your best features – you must love all of it. If you reject any part of you, you are ultimately rejecting yourself. This rejection of the self is expressed in the cells in a negative way, whereas when you accept and love every part of you, your cells feel loved, appreciated and valued, and they act accordingly.

I realise that this might sound almost too simple to be believable, but it is true. Your body mirrors what is going on in your mind, and your cells mirror what you feel about yourself by behaving in a way that matches the feeling.

Focus on the positives

In order to have healthy cells, you need a healthy attitude about yourself, so we are going to begin the process by focusing on all the positive things about you. We are often uncomfortable focusing on what is good about ourselves and quick to focus on what we think is wrong with us. In fact many people seem to feel easier criticising themselves than praising themselves, saying, 'I look awful in this', 'I look old, fat, tired . . .', and so on, yet when they are given a compliment they can actually become uncomfortable; for example:

Compliment	What you might say
'You look nice.'	'What? In this old thing?'
'Your hair looks nice.'	'No, it can't do – it needs washing.'
'That's a nice dress.'	'Oh, it's so old. I've had it for years.'
'You did really well today.'	'Oh it was nothing really.'

Isn't it odd that running yourself down is easy and familiar, and praising yourself feels uncomfortable and unfamiliar? It is unnatural to criticise yourself, because criticism withers people, whereas praise makes them grow. We must learn to take compliments more easily. This will only happen if we give ourselves more compliments and begin to see all the good things that are part of us, not the opposite. We can always find whatever we look for. If you look for what is negative about yourself you can find something, and if you look for what is positive you can find something. You must learn to look for what is good and positive about you, about your appearance, your age and your character.

It is lovely to be given a compliment and it can make us feel great when someone says something nice about us; however, there is a big difference between liking compliments and actually needing them in order to feel good about ourselves. If you always need compliments it will make you needy, which is not a good state to be in. Giving yourself compliments regularly will move you to a much better and healthier state of mind and well-being.

Give yourself a lot of compliments and praise yourself a lot – it will raise your self-esteem massively. Compliment people around you as well, because not only will it make them feel good, but it will also have a good effect on you. One of the most rapid and easiest ways to raise your self-esteem is to raise the self-esteem of others, to praise and compliment others. Obviously, it must be genuine, but it is so easy to find something nice to say about someone else, and your own self-esteem will grow in the most beneficial way when you start doing this. Studies show that self-praise has the same effect as receiving praise from others, so if your boss never says 'you did a great job', say it to yourself. If your partner does not tell you enough that you are lovely and loveable, tell yourself this on a regular basis.

The old school of thought said that praising people makes them big headed and arrogant, whereas criticism stops them from getting above themselves. This is not true at all. Criticism defeats people, whereas praise makes them grow, so praise more and criticise less, especially yourself. You can only change yourself. This book is about you making changes for you, so praise yourself more and criticise yourself less. Stop saying, 'Oh, I'm so stupid', 'I can't believe I did that', 'I'm an idiot', 'I'm an old fool', 'I look horrible', 'I'm too fat', 'I'm too old.' You must give up this negative self-criticism and instead find out all the good things about you and focus on them.

If you occasionally find yourself saying, 'I did something stupid', change it to 'I made a mistake'. We all make mistakes, and if you lapse into criticising yourself, just decide not to believe it.

I do this if I get lost on a journey or I get delayed – it is so easy to say, 'I can't believe I didn't look up the journey before I left' or 'I'm so stupid for not leaving earlier.' Although I make a point of not speaking to myself like that, if I do, I decide not to believe what I am saying and instead I tell myself it is OK to get lost, it's all right to be late occasionally. I don't allow myself to believe any pointless criticism, including my own, although constructive criticism has a value.

Of course, you may have experiences of people who seem very arrogant and full of themselves and this has put you off the idea of self-praise; however, people who come across as truly arrogant usually don't actually believe in themselves very much at all. They are the opposite end of the same scale of people who lack confidence, so they put on a show of confidence, not just to convince others but to convince themselves.

People who truly like themselves have no need to do this. You can be quietly confident, you can radiate inner confidence, you can believe in yourself and you can do all of this for your own benefit. If you believe you are ageless, beautiful and wonderful, you won't feel the need to convince others of the same – it just won't be necessary. Yet, by putting a higher value on yourself, you will automatically increase the value that other people have of you. If you increase your self-image, others will too. The most important and the most powerful words you will ever hear are the words you say to yourself and believe. The most important opinion for you is your opinion.

I learned long ago that the best thing to do is to pay no attention to flaws, because no one else notices them – or at least notices them to the degree that you do. People tend to see us the way we see ourselves, they pick up the way we feel about ourselves because our self-image reflects from us to the people we are around, who then reflect it back to us. If you cease to notice minor flaws, no one else will pay them much attention either, but if you go on and on about them, you only draw attention to something you want to go unnoticed.

Ignore others' criticism

Sometimes we dislike a part of ourselves for no valid reason. When I was younger I had a real complex about my legs. They were so skinny, and all the boys at school used to call me twiglet because I guess that's what they thought my legs looked like. Luckily, my grandmother told me it was a compliment, so it bothered me a little less, although out of school I never ever wore skirts and I lived in trousers. I was dating a guy from outside my school when I was 16 and worked as a waitress in a restaurant on a Saturday. One day he unexpectedly came in to see me and I remember standing behind a table because I was so determined he would not see my legs, since a skirt was part of the uniform. I went on and on about how thin they were, and he picked up my belief system and eventually agreed with me.

I'm not sure when I began to think differently, but I do remember my next boyfriend telling me I had the best legs he had ever seen. When I was an exercise teacher, many of the girls in my class used to say, 'If I do your class can I get legs like yours?' I had an article written about me in *Marie Claire* and they very nicely wrote 'Marisa Peer has the kind of legs that make you ponder on life's injustices.'

Somewhere in between hating my legs and being extremely self-conscious of them I grew to love them and see them as an asset, and many times I have been told I have wonderful legs. This wasn't because they changed as I got older – they are still exactly the same legs, but I felt differently about them. My legs have never changed shape or size, but I have changed from hating them and feeling self-conscious and embarrassed about them to loving them.

When you are able to do this about every part of your body, you will feel so different, and this different expression and feeling about yourself will cause your cells to pick up the positive feelings about you and thrive instead of wither.

Sometimes though, I still get told my legs are too skinny, but once I had begun to like them I didn't really care what anyone else said, because I was happy with them and had accepted them. I was crossing the road in London once and a man came up to me and said, 'Your legs are like matchsticks.' I was able to burst out laughing and reply, 'Your brain is made of the same material.' Only unattractive men have come up to me to tell me my legs are too thin. It is interesting and amazing that they seem to feel it is OK to comment on my body, but I have come to realise that the people who criticise us always have the most criticism reserved for themselves.

WHAT MAKES PEOPLE CRITICAL?

Critical people simply reflect their own self-criticism. It is as if they have to make everyone else aware of any faults or flaws so that they don't feel alone in their negative self-judgement; they seem to need us all to feel as bad about part of ourselves as they secretly do about themselves, then they can feel more comfortable. It seems to be something about safety in numbers. Critical people have the most criticism reserved for themselves, so when they criticise someone else, they are really describing their own world and talking in a paradox. Maxim Gorky (1868–1936) said, 'A miserable man must find a more miserable man then he is happy.'

If you are around people who criticise you, refuse to absorb it. Only people who feel mediocre criticise – superior people praise. As you cease to criticise yourself and others you will feel quite different, and your cells will become a real and physical expression of this different and positive feeling. It helps to remind yourself, and the critic, that critical people who focus on other people's flaws are usually so aware of their own that they feel deep down that they are not good enough. They seem to need to make everyone else aware of their own flaws so that others too will feel not good enough. That way, they can then keep the critics company.

If they feel inadequate, and almost all critical people do, then they will want you to feel inadequate too. They may only feel equal to you if they criticise you. Critical people, who feel inadequate, know that the only way they can balance this is to diminish you or to elevate themselves, but either behaviour simply highlights their own feelings of inadequacy.

Fashions influence us

People are very easily influenced – fashions show us that. We don't feel comfortable wearing something that is judged as unfashionable or dated, although in its moment of fashion we loved it. Once it is judged to be no longer fashionable, however, we are embarrassed to be seen in the garment. Of course, the clothing itself hasn't changed, but we have changed our opinion and become influenced by fashion. We are also very influenced by fashions, not just in clothes but in furniture, food, music, and so on, as well. We are all easily influenced, but unaware that we have the power to influence how we feel about ourselves and, consequently, how everyone else feels about us.

Learn to love yourself

When I was teaching exercise classes in Chicago, one of my fellow teachers was small and quite muscular and yet she had a fantastic body image. She would always say during her class, 'I love my legs. They are strong and they carry me around. They are so good to me. I love my body, because it takes care of me so well.' She never compared herself to anyone or said, 'I wish I looked like that.' She didn't ever complain about her body, but always praised it and acknowledged it; she accepted herself and taught herself to feel great about her looks and herself. She obviously made an impression on me, because I have never forgotten her.

I also have a friend who has the most amazing, perfect body. I asked her once what it was like to have such a body, since I imagined it must be wonderful and that she would be uninhibited and free of all complexes. I assumed she would feel lucky and proud. Certainly, all her friends envied her. She answered, 'My body is a curse to me, and it always has been. Men stare at me and make me feel uncomfortable. They only want to get to know me because they love my body – and I hate it.'

I was stunned by her response and learned a lot from it. I have since noticed how many of my most attractive clients (some of them truly beautiful models and actresses) have as many, if not more, complexes about how they look than the plainer ones who want to lose weight or look better. Greta Scacchi recently said that she was delighted to lose her looks, because she could finally go to the supermarket without men leering at her. She said she has never been happier and would not want her previous good looks back.

My unhappy clients who are models are always comparing themselves to someone else whom they see as prettier or younger. It is such a waste. You cannot compare yourself with anyone, because you are unique. Beauty is not just in the eye of the beholder – it is in our eyes. How we see ourselves is reflected to the world. We can choose to see ourselves in a positive light and so will everyone else. Our partners don't really care if we are a few pounds overweight – they probably don't even notice – but if you go on about it they will notice and may begin to feel about it the way you feel about it. If you share your life with people who criticise your appearance, remind yourself that they are insecure about themselves. By all means make changes that will allow you to feel better, but do it for you.

You can change any belief about yourself – you don't have to look like a model to appreciate yourself. You don't have to be young to have value. Real beauty comes from within. Learn to love every bit of yourself and see a value in your body. Wrinkles are character lines, stretch marks left by being lucky enough to have children. I worked with a model who was unable to have a baby. She told me, 'I would be prepared to have a body covered in stretch marks from head to foot and would willingly sacrifice my figure permanently in order to have a baby. I don't care what I look like. I would trade all of this now if I could only have a baby. My looks can never give me the pleasure that having a child of my own could.'

Don't get caught in the trap of saying, 'I hate my nose/stom-ach/thighs/face.' If you can change some body parts through diet and exercise, by all means do that, but if you can't change a part of yourself, accept it and look for some positive aspects of it. The worst thing we can do is to fall into the trap of believing and saying, 'I can't accept it and I can't change it. I hate this part of me and I can't do anything about it.'

Barbra Streisand has a larger nose, which has never detracted from her beauty. All around us are examples of men and women who are not at all perfect but who believe in themselves with such conviction that we do as well. The singer Gabrielle wore an eye patch, but that has not stopped her becoming a famous pop singer. Seal has very visible scars on his face, but women find him gorgeous. Both Trudie Styler and the actress Tina Fey have very visible scars on their face. Amanda Redman has a deeply scarred arm, as does the supermodel Padma Lakshmi.

When my little girl was five, she was in the bath and said to me, 'Mummy, I hate my hair. It's too curly. I hate my mouth and I hate my body.' I couldn't believe that my baby, who has always been brought up around positive thinking, had already begun to have such a negative body image. Her two best friends were Japanese and I had told them how pretty they were and what beautiful shiny straight hair they had. When I took them out, people would often say how pretty and well behaved they were, and my daughter decided she wanted to be like her friends and was comparing herself to them unfavourably.

I said to her, 'Tell me what you *do* like about you first. Let's talk about what you love about you.' And she reeled off a list of things, starting with her eyes, her teeth, her smile, her skin and she immediately began to feel better about herself. As the list got longer she forgot to be negative.

When she would say, 'Mummy, do I look pretty in this?' I always said, 'What do you think you look like?' And she always replied, 'Oh I think I look gorgeous', and I would tell her that is what counts, what you think you look like matters most of all, but I would tell her she's gorgeous too – I want her to believe in herself.

She once came home from school and said, 'A boy in my class said I am ugly', and so I asked her, 'Do you think you are ugly?' She looked at me and said, 'No, I know I am not ugly.' So then I asked her how she knew she wasn't ugly and she told me, and then I asked her why she would pay any attention to someone else who was only trying to upset her. We must all learn to value our own opinions and to place more on them than on the opinions of someone else who may not have our best interests at heart.

When I was little, my relatives all used to say, 'Aren't you tall? Aren't your feet big?' and I remember so much longing to be petite, because they didn't say, 'Aren't you tall?' in a positive way. It's so easy to get a complex. In fact, I love being tall, and my feet are size five, but when I was nine I worried that I would grow into a giant because people commented on my height in a way that made me feel negative about it and conscious of it.

I refused to have my photograph taken for years, because I hated the way I looked. Years later when I looked at photos of myself as a child I was surprised that I was cute, because I felt ugly at the time, but of course these feelings weren't based on anything real or rational. They very rarely are. I see this with so many of my clients who have a very negative self-image when they look absolutely fine, and although I could tell them they look wonderful, my job is to make them absolutely believe and feel they look wonderful, that they *are* wonderful and that they are unique and cannot be compared to anyone else.

If we feel negative and get criticised, it can hurt. If we feel positive, we can let it go.

When I was appearing on television the *Mirror* newspaper wrote that I had a moustache and should shave it off. I know I don't have one and that it was just bad lighting, so I did not let that affect me, and some weeks later they wrote about me again, but this time were very complimentary.

Block negative criticism

One of the best lessons I ever learned, which has helped me beyond measure, was not to let in negative criticism. The most important thing is to like yourself, to learn to love every part of yourself. We cannot amputate parts of ourselves. We have to learn to accept them and look for the positive. In this section you are going to acknowledge yourself in the most positive way, to focus on all the things you like about yourself and to make this list longer and much more significant than any negative list you may have. We will do this with your looks, your age and your personality.

At the end of this section, you are going to make a list of all the good things about you. As you make this list, remember that every cell of your body hears and responds to the words and feelings you have about yourself. The more you criticise your body, the more despondent it becomes, and the more you praise it, the more it reacts to your praise. If you praise your body more and more, it will literally change and function much better, as well as looking and feeling better.

Feel you are a miracle

You have a mind within each and every one of your trillions of body cells, and these cells, unlike brain cells, have no ability to doubt what you tell them; they accept your words and opinions as the absolute truth. By making your words, opinions and thoughts more and more positive, you can change your emotional and physical body. Happy thoughts quite literally make happy cells. When you are feeling happy and feeling good about yourself, every cell in your body is an expression of this feeling. When you are feeling dissatisfied with yourself, every cell in your body is an expression of this feeling too.

As you tell your body and yourself how wonderful you look, how wonderful your body is at taking care of you, at performing daily miracles that keep you alive, your body will physically respond to these words in the most positive way.

The UK private healthcare agency BUPA ran a series of very successful adverts that focused on all the miracles of the human body. The heading of each advert was 'You are a miracle. We want to keep you that way.' You are indeed a miracle – the human body does so many amazing things, and by thinking this way, by focusing on the wonderful things your body does for you daily, and by thanking it and acknowledging it instead of criticising it, your body will respond to you and you can remain a miracle and look, feel and remain younger throughout your life.

Imagine if your body was a person – how do you think it would feel if you said, 'I hate my body', or 'How could anyone love this old body', or 'I hate my stomach/legs' on a regular basis? It would feel despondent and would feel like giving up and not bothering, since it is so unappreciated. Your cells would become a physical expression of despondency. This can, and does, happen within the body – the more you love your body, the more loveable it will become to you, and the more it will respond to you.

We have receptor sites in the body, including the liver, kidneys, bone marrow and immune system, that respond to our thoughts, so a form of communication or interplay is always going on between the mind and the body. When you feel despair, or if you hate parts of yourself, your body responds to this feeling of giving up by giving up with you, by not bothering to make the healing chemicals you need to thrive, because your body has to express the same despair that is going on silently in your mind.

Love makes you strong, healthy and young

You are making a very different body when you are happy or feeling joy. You are also making a very different body when you are at peace with yourself. Your body chemistry or biochemistry will be very different from that of someone who is unhappy with themselves.

Joan Borysenko, a cell biologist at Tufts University, researched the power of the mind to heal and wrote about the very real power our mind has to change cells. She documented many of the experiments that I refer to. Bernie Siegal gives a great example of this in his book *Love, Medicine and Miracles* when he talks about the tests that have proved lovers are more resistant to poison, because their immune system is so good. The tests prove the power that feeling loved has on the body, especially the immune system. In the state of being loved we feel cherished, valued and appreciated, and our body literally responds to that feeling.

Good relationships always help us. That feeling of being loved is so important, which is why people who have a good relationship with themselves generally live longer and are healthier. From today, you are going to have a good relationship with yourself and to cherish, value and appreciate yourself.

Start now to love your body, to love everything about it, and you will very quickly notice how much better it performs for you. Begin to credit your body rather than discredit it; instead of complaining about what it won't or hasn't done, see all the excellent things it does for you. As you re-evaluate your body in a positive way, it will respond positively to this re-evaluation.

I also recommend that you take a few moments and apologise to your body for all the negative things you have thought and said about it and make a decision not to do this anymore.

Exercise 15: Appreciate your body

1   Remember every compliment you have ever been given for what you are, what you do, how you look, and so on. Let your mind go back over the years and remember all the nice things people have said about you. Write out every one of these compliments.

2   Now add to the list by complimenting yourself on how you look.

3   Work through your body from head to toe, complimenting yourself on your hair, your eyes, your skin, your smile, your body, the way you move, how nice you always smell, how infectious your laugh is, and so on.

▶

4   Thank your body for looking after you and for taking care of you so well.

5   Repeat these statements to yourself and, as you do, feel and imagine your body getting the message.

6   As you make each statement out loud, feel as if it is true right now.

7   Repeat the following statements out loud, and as you say each one, *feel* that it is all true at this moment:

a   My body is *ageless*.

b   My body is *graceful*.

c   I have shiny, bright, lovely *eyes*, and they see the beauty in me and in everyone else.

d   My *hair* is shiny, glossy and healthy, and it always smells lovely.

e   My *teeth* allow me to eat anything I wish.

f   I have a beautiful *smile*.

g   My *skin* is soft and lovely to touch.

h   My *hands* are such an asset to me; what would I do without them?

i   My *body* is a miracle: it digests food, combines it with oxygen from the air I breathe and uses it to build the perfect body for me.

j   I love my body. I love *myself*.

k   My *memory* is great. I can remember so many things. I have a wonderful mind.

▶

l   I have a great *heart*, powerful *lungs*, *muscles* that take care of me, a good *nervous system*, a strong *immune system* and *legs* that take me anywhere I want to go.

m   I am a *wonderful* dancer.

n   I have a *beautiful* voice.

o   People love me because *I am me*.

p   I am *loveable*, I am enough and I always will be enough, and I will always be loveable.

Add any other statements to your list that are applicable to you.

As you appreciate your body, it will become more appreciable to you, so get in to the habit of appreciating yourself every day.

Summary – Step Nine

Let's recap all you have learned in this step.

- You have learned all about your cells and the role they play in ageing.
- You have learned that you have the power and ability to talk to your cells as easily as you might talk to a friend, to give your cells clear instructions in the way you want them to behave and to have that behaviour begin. You now have a programme for cellular regeneration that you can listen to or refer to daily.
- You have learned what happens when you criticise yourself

or hate parts of yourself and the very real and negative effect
this has on your body.

- You have learned how to understand and deal with critical
  people.
- You have learned to reclaim yourself as a beautiful and
  wonderful person.
- You have learned that the most important compliments and
  opinions are your opinions about yourself and that you have
  full power to influence them in a truly positive way

'Whatever you can do, or dream, you can, begin it.
Boldness has genius, magic and power in it.
Begin it now'

Attributed to Johann Wolfgang von Goethe
(1749–1832)

Change Your Lifestyle and Habits

'You either have to be part of the solution, or you're going to be part of the problem'

Eldridge Cleaver (1935–98)

Welcome to the last step of my programme, which is destined to make you feel and look years younger. Since beginning to read this book you have done some powerful work to change your concept of ageing and to change the way you are ageing. You have changed your thoughts, your beliefs, your language and your physiology. Now we are going to cover changing your lifestyle and changing some of your habits. Lifestyle is very important, and making some simple changes to it can increase your life by at least 10 years, and can even add up to 30 years to your life. Your body can quite literally become younger instead of becoming older, if you treat it the right way.

I have spent most of this book focusing on changing your thinking, your attitudes and your beliefs, and I have told you numerous times by now that that is the most important thing of all, that making changes in what you think and believe can and will change how you age. Now we are moving on to another equally important section of the book. If you believed up until now that all you had to do was change your thinking and you feel disappointed that you have to make lifestyle changes as well, let me reassure you. Changing your thinking is the most important step, which is why it is Step One. Does that mean that in theory you could think positively, live a destructive lifestyle and stay younger? In theory you may very well be able to do this, and lots of people such as Chuck Berry and Keith Richards have, but you bought this book because you want to become younger, and you want to hold on to looking and feeling younger than you are chronologically, throughout your life. If you are serious about wanting to become younger, to live longer, and to look and feel younger at any age (and it is such a great subject to be serious about), then it is absolutely worth making lifestyle changes as well, especially since the ones in this book are easy to make.

If you want to become younger, and you have followed all the earlier steps, but you live on junk food, you never exercise and you sleep in close proximity to a lot of electrical equipment (explained on page 243), you will deny yourself the full and wonderful results you could achieve. Why settle for anything less than results of 100 per cent?

I am very aware that many programmes that promote lifestyle changes fail because they are too rigid and they sell you a lifestyle that you may not be able to maintain. With this in mind I have developed a chapter of easy lifestyle changes that will give you a lot of choice, a lot of flexibility and a lot of say in the changes you make.

Get into the right habits

Ninety-five per cent of what we do is habit and is automatic, so it follows that changing even some of these habits will make a big impact on your ability to age successfully. What you begin and repeat over and over will become a new habit, a habit that has lasting and visible benefits. By taking action today, you can make anti-ageing a new habit and part of a new and enriching lifestyle for you.

It is important not to get stuck in a rut or an outdated routine, because that in itself is very ageing. If you want to stay young, learn something new. Make variety your best friend and routine your enemy. Humans can learn something new at any age, because they have the ability to be flexible in attitudes and beliefs. You don't even need to work at eliminating old habits – you can simply replace them with new ones instead.

Doing something as simple as cleaning your teeth with your non-dominant hand (the left for most of us) and using the less-dominant hand to change channels on the TV or to dial telephone numbers, or to use a spoon or hold a cup teaches your brain something new, strengthening neuron connections and creating new ones. Going up the stairs starting with the non-dominant leg (usually the left) has the same effect. Any brain exercises can stave off brain degeneration while also reversing memory loss and improving mental agility.

Stimulation keeps your brain engaged and growing. Doing something different deepens and creates new brain pathways.

Over the next few pages you will discover the anti-ageing properties of diet, vitamins, supplements, exercise and skin brushing. Even the way you sleep, and the amount of electricity you are sleeping close to, is relevant. I have written each section in a way that gives you masses of choice – you can choose which wonder-foods to include in your diet, and which vitamins and supplements to take. It's a form of healthy pick-and-mix. You will be given a list of things that will allow you to maintain good digestion, which is strongly linked to good ageing, and a list that shows you how to limit easily and effectively the amount of electricity your body is exposed to, especially when you sleep, as well as learning the anti-ageing properties of correct sleep.

You will also learn the benefits of exercise in limiting bone and muscle loss while maintaining agility, energy and hormone levels, and you will learn the wonderful and immediate benefits of skin brushing. It's so important that you enter into these with the belief and commitment that you are going to make wonderful changes and that this change is one you will look back on as significant. From this point forward, you will be taking action that will allow you to become younger and live longer and more healthily.

Diet and ageing

'To lengthen thy life, lessen thy meals'

Benjamin Franklin (1706–90)

We are what we eat – and this is especially true with ageing. If you want to look and feel fabulous throughout your life, you need to pay attention to what you eat, and this becomes more important as you get older, because every single atom in your body is fuelled by food. I want to introduce you to what I call nature's super-foods or wonder-foods, foods that if included in your diet will give you the vitamins, the super-nutrition and the antioxidants that will allow you to successfully fight ageing.

Antioxidants are nutrients, vitamins C and E and beta-carotene. They are found in fruit, vegetables, nuts and seeds. Antioxidants are the body's defence against free radicals and free-radical damage. Free radicals are highly reactive molecules that surge through the body causing oxidization damage to all kinds of cells. They damage healthy genes and cells, and are linked to the onset of ageing, as well as to cancer and heart disease. Anti-oxidants offer protection against free radicals. Foods that contain beta-carotene and vitamins C and E are known as free-radical scavengers. As we saw earlier, scientists at the Biology of Aging Program at the National Institute on Aging in Maryland, USA, believe we could live to 120 years old if we could prevent the molecular damage occurring in our cells.

For many people, sticking to a particular eating regime is difficult, especially if they have to prepare food for family members
who don't share their enthusiasm for healthy eating, or if their
business involves a lot of entertaining or eating out. Many
healthy-eating plans fail because they are too rigid and inflexible,
so they can be difficult to stick with, causing people to think, 'I
can't do this properly, so I might as well not do it at all.'

I am going to show you all the foods that truly are nature's best
and I recommend that you include them in your diet. Those
marked with an asterisk are the best of all. If you include as many
of these foods as possible into your weekly eating plan, you will
reap the benefits.

This will allow you to put together an eating plan that suits
you, is easy to stick to and that adapts well to eating out and
catering for others. You can easily include this eating plan while
travelling and for packed lunches – in fact, you can include it
wherever you go.

This list is not meant to replace your diet but to help you
ensure that you always include the foods within it. You could
exist very healthily on this diet alone, but you don't have to. The
more of these foods you include, the healthier you will be. If you
eat predominately healthy food, your body can cope with you
eating unhealthy food occasionally. Certainly, making changes,
like replacing margarine with olive oil, and giving up hydrogenated oils, will assist you to look and feel your best because
hydrogenated fats can accelerate oxygen-based damage to cells. It
has been said that just cutting out all hydrogenated fats or trans-
fats (used in margarines and many processed foods) as well as
cutting out artificial sweeteners can add 16 years to your lifespan.

Cutting calories will have the same effect, but only if you eat
food that is nourishing. We can live 50 per cent longer on a lean
diet. Tests have been done on mice, rats, monkeys and squirrels
showing that if their calorie intake is reduced they live 50 per cent
longer, have less oxygen-based damage to their cells, and delay the
onset of disease. It is not a question of under-eating but of eating

food that is healthy, eating much less sugar and starch and more lean protein and vegetables. Eating this way will cause you to consume fewer calories naturally, but you don't have to feel hungry or go hungry, the stress of that is not recommended or anti-ageing.

In alphabetical order, here is the list of wonder-foods that are essential to anti-ageing:

Apples are rich in oxygen. The skins contain pectin, which is a setting agent and is beneficial if you have an upset stomach. Pectin – an anti-cholesterol agent – can lower cholesterol and reduce blood pressure. Pectin also helps rid the body of metals, which is vital if we are to fight ageing. Apples contain phyto-estrogens, substances found in plants that may be able to prevent harmful oestrogens from causing breast cancer. Apples contain magnesium, which can stop sugar cravings.

Apricots are part of the staple diet of the Hunza people, who routinely seem to live into their hundredth year. Dried apricots are excellent too, but only if they aren't coated in preservatives and sulphur. The black dried apricots from Turkey, and Hunza apricots, are the best. Apricots contain lycopene and beta-carotene, which protect against age-related cell damage and oxidation of proteins and fats, while boosting the immune system.

Asparagus is one of the best sources of folic acid, which may help prevent strokes and reduce the risk of breast and colon cancer. It's also loaded with glutathione, which fights premature ageing by repairing damage to the DNA and boosting immunity.

* **Avocado** This is one of the best foods of all. It is packed with vitamins, including vitamin E, minerals and antioxidants. It has more potassium than bananas (potassium lowers blood pressure and reduces high sodium levels). It is rich in glutathione, which protects the body from toxins, helps to neutralise the bad fat that damages our bodies, and is the most powerful antioxidant, fighting the free-radical damage to cells that is a major cause of all ageing. Some studies from the US have shown that people with the highest levels of glutathione had lower blood pressure and lower cholesterol and were generally leaner and healthier. Research studies show that when mosquitoes deficient in glutathione were given the correct amount, their lifespan increased by 40 per cent. Avocados are high in the good fat that the body needs and makes excellent use of. They also contain oleic acid, which helps to transform memories from short term to long term. You can safely eat an avocado every day. They have been proven to lower and improve blood cholesterol. Avocado mashed up and spread over the face, then allowed to dry and washed off afterwards, makes an excellent face pack and is restoring for tired, stressed skin.

* **Beetroot** is wonderful for the endocrine system; it's restorative for the liver and is an anti-cancer food. Lightly cooked beetroot is tasty in salads. Raw beetroot is excellent juiced into carrot or carrot and apple juice, using about a quarter of the beetroot with the remaining juice ingredients. Roasted beets are a great alternative to roast potatoes.

Berries All the red, black and blue berries are crammed full of antioxidants and quercetin, which fight ageing. Strawberries are full of iodine and pectin, and seem to fight cancer in older people. Blueberries and cranberries are good for urinary tract infections, but don't add sugar to them, as sugar feeds infection. As with all produce, buy organic berries if you can, or ensure that you wash them really well. Some cooks believe that washing strawberries spoils the flavour, but you must wash fruit or you will ingest all the pesticides and chemicals that damage cells and accelerate ageing.

* **Broccoli** is truly a super-food. It deserves to be in the top ten of all foods, as it contains properties that fight bone loss and cancer. Broccoli contains sulphoraphane, which boosts anti-cancer enzymes. A 100g (3½oz) portion of broccoli has 205mg of calcium – more than any other vegetable. It is also rich in iron and

folic acid. Broccoli contains masses of antioxidants, including vitamin C, beta-carotene, glutathione (which neutralises bad fats), quercetin and potassium. Broccoli also contains chromium and helps rid the body of the harmful type of oestrogen that can cause cancer, while quercetin protects against heart disease and heart attacks.[10] Purple sprouting broccoli is even better as it contains iron, calcium and folic acid. All types of broccoli boost the immune system.

Brazil nuts, still in their shell, are full of selenium, which is essential for anti-ageing.[11] Each Brazil nut, straight from the shell, contains about 100mcg of selenium – more than in most selenium tablets. Other food sources of selenium are sunflower seeds, garlic and seafood. You don't need more than 200mcg a day, and having two Brazil nuts daily, or every other day, will give you all the selenium you need. If you eat the other selenium-rich foods mentioned, one Brazil nut daily or every other day is enough. Brazil nuts purchased shelled have much less selenium and can be rancid if they have been stored for too long. Chocolate-coated Brazil nuts, sadly, don't count at all.

* **Carrots** lower blood cholesterol. The orange pigment in carrots boosts immune function and protects against cancer and strokes. The high levels of vitamin A in carrots are excellent for maintaining healthy skin, and the alpha-carotene they contain may help prevent cardiovascular disease. Carrots really are good for your eyesight, as the beta-carotene contained in them will protect the eyes from eye-related diseases that often occur with ageing.

* **Cabbage** Savoy cabbage is the best and is full of antioxidants. All cabbages have anti-cancer properties and are rich in potassium. Like broccoli, cabbage can help rid the body of the harmful oestrogens that can cause breast cancer. Oestrogen in excessive amounts can alter cell structures and may lead to breast cancer. Cabbage contains indoles that help detoxify the body.[12] Red cabbage is also excellent.

* **Eggs** are the most complete food on the planet after breast milk, and contain everything to sustain life. They are a true wonder-food. Eggs are a great source of lutein, which protects against macular eye degeneration (the most common cause of blindness in the UK, and as there is no cure and only limited treatment for it, prevention is vital). Eggs contain sulphur, which protects against the harmful effect of being over-exposed to electromagnetic fields – there is about 65mg of sulphur in each egg. They are rich in vitamins A, B, D and E, and contain zinc, iron, lecithin, selenium, trace minerals and every amino acid the body needs. Many athletes swear by the properties of egg yolks, especially when training or competing. You can safely eat eggs every single day. A beaten egg applied to the face and allowed to dry, then washed off, has a tightening, lifting effect and although the results are temporary and last only for about 24 hours, it has been used for centuries as a beauty treatment; it was used by the ancient Egyptians and was a favourite routine of film stars in the 20th century, as it made them look years younger.

* **Fish** Omega-3 oils are found in salmon, tuna, mackerel, sardines, herrings and, to a lesser degree, in halibut, cod and haddock. These same fish are also full of antioxidants, including selenium and co-enzyme Q_{10} (CoQ_{10}). Omega-3 fatty acids may have a direct effect on extending the lifespan of cells. They may slow down damage to DNA and can protect against inflammation and other ageing processes. Omega-3 oils are known as essential oils and they are essential for a reason: every part of our body and brain needs them. Omega-3 oils are able to offer cells protection against ageing because they have blood-thinning properties that protect arteries and lower blood pressure. They also have anti-inflammatory properties and can protect against heart attacks, strokes and some cancers, while improving joint mobility. Your brain is mostly made of fat and 60 per cent of this fat consists of essential fatty acids.

The vital ingredients in fish oil are EPA and DHA, which are the essential fatty acids that the body needs and cannot make for itself.

You can only get these essential fatty acids by including fish or fish oils in your diet. DHA is needed to make the nerve connections between brain cells and the cell membranes of brain tissue, and it is also essential for vision and memory. Low levels of DHA are associated with poor mental performance and depression.

The Omega-3 oils can balance out high amounts of Omega-6 fatty acids, which can be as bad as Omega-3 is good. Omega-6 is found in bad fats that damage our cells. Omega-3 oils have been proven to reverse a substantial amount of this damage.

People in Japan, who on average live far longer than people in the West, eat 200 per cent more fish than we do. Seafood is high in magnesium. Bony fish in particular – such as salmon and sardines – is full of calcium. According to Danish research, Omega-3 in fish oils may help pregnant mothers carry their babies to full term and may be able to prolong gestation in mothers likely to give birth prematurely, because it shifts the balance of production of prostaglandins involved in parturition.

* **Flaxseeds (milled)** are a good plant source of Omega-3 and vitamin E – especially useful for vegans. The oil from flaxseeds, which are also known as linseeds, has long been associated with a long and healthy life and was used as a therapeutic remedy in ancient Greece and Rome. The essential fatty acids (EFAs) in flaxseeds are used by the body for cell oxygenation, and they promote a healthy immune system. The body cannot produce EFAs, so they must be supplied by food. Flaxseed oil has a natural detoxifying effect on the body and is known traditionally as 'super-skin nutrition', which can prevent drying and flaking skin. The oil can be eaten straight from a spoon or used as a salad dressing, but don't cook with it or you will destroy its benefits. Ground or milled flaxseeds are also easy to take sprinkled over food. Because they don't have much of a flavour, they can be added to yoghurt, soups, salads or any dishes after cooking. Flaxseeds have a well-deserved reputation as being an excellent, safe and natural remedy for constipation (which is bad for your skin), drawing toxins out of the body.

* **Garlic** helps to reduce fat. German studies show that the triglyceride level in a person who had eaten garlic was 35 per cent lower than a person who had not (high triglyceride levels indicate an elevated risk of stroke). Garlic also helps to maintain circulation to the skin, and this supply of oxygenated blood helps the skin, hair and nails to stay strong and healthy. It also contains quercetin and 400 chemicals, including many antioxidants. It is a natural antibiotic and decongestant, and it reduces cholesterol and blood pressure while boosting the immune system.[13]

* **Ginger** has an ability to deter blood clots, due to the gingerol, an anti-coagulant and blood thinner, contained within it. It is similar to aspirin, but far preferable, since it won't irritate your stomach. Ginger is excellent at reversing signs of hearing loss and arthritis; it also helps with nausea during travel and pregnancy, and alleviates stomach distension as well as assisting digestion. It has been used in China for over 2,000 years and is used in 50 per cent of all oriental prescriptions.

You don't need to take much ginger at all – it can be taken in capsule form, but it is also a great ingredient to cook with, especially in stir-fried vegetables, fish or chicken dishes. I make a flask of ginger tea using fresh root ginger and lemon juice; sometimes I add a stick of cinnamon and a touch of honey. It makes a very soothing drink if you have a sore throat – and it tastes delicious.[14]

* **Grapes** If you have a sweet tooth, small red grapes are one of the sweetest fruits around and do an excellent job of curtailing the craving. You will find that once you eat less sugar it becomes too sweet and begins to lose its appeal. Your body likes and asks for what you give it all the time. The less sugar you consume, the less your body will want it. I used to have a sweet tooth and would never have believed this myself, but it's true. With milk chocolate and other refined sugars, the more you get a taste for it the more you want. Switching to fruit is the best thing, if you plan to age well. Refined sugar isn't a food but a chemical; it's produced in a refinery like petrol and has no sell-by-date, because it never, ever decomposes. Sugar dramatically ages your skin, because it attaches to collagen making the skin stiff, jowly and rigid, and making wrinkles more defined.

Red grapes are better for you than green, because all the antioxidants in grapes (and they contain at least 20) are in the skin. The deeper the hue of the skin, the more antioxidants there are. The antioxidants in grapes have an anti-clogging ability and do great work for our arteries; the skin of red grapes also contains a cholesterol-lowering ingredient.[15] A handful daily is enough as they are a high-sugar fruit.

Honey Organic cold-pressed honey is a wonder-food and was used by the ancient Egyptians as a common remedy for a variety of ailments. Honey has antiseptic healing properties and has been used to treat wounds by the ancient Greeks, Romans and Chinese, among others. It was even used in the First World War as an anti-septic. It seems to cause bacteria to disintegrate and has been proven to kill infectious organisms.

Because honey is a form of sugar, you need only take a tiny amount of it, no more than half a teaspoon a day. Honey put onto wounds can have a very healing effect, and honey applied to the face is a good form of face mask and helpful for removing old cells, which will dull the complexion.

Many tribes of people who live to 100 years or more, yet remain youthful, eat diets rich in bee pollen and propolis. Propolis is the substance made by bees to seal the hive together, protecting it from the outer environment and creating a totally sterile environment. Propolis produces the autoimmune system for the hive and is antibiotic, antiviral and antifungal. Propolis is also loaded with amino acids, vitamins, minerals and bioflavonoids, which are involved in the healing process. You can take propolis as a supplement. It has been found to be effective for colds, flu, many viruses, arthritis and rheumatic problems. The term 'cold-pressed' means that the product has not been heat treated, which causes it to lose its essential vitamins, so don't put honey or propolis in hot drinks or cook with it.

Legumes (pulses) and grains Sprouted grains, millet, buckwheat, barley and lentils are all foods high in antioxidants, magnesium, and vitamins B and E, and they are a good source of protein. They contain saponins, which can slow the growth of tumours. They also contain selenium, potassium, calcium, iron and zinc. Barley has antiviral and anti-cancer properties and is high in antioxidants. Millet is rich in protein, iron, potassium, magnesium and minerals that protect against heart disease. Buckwheat, which is actually not a type of wheat, is full of protein and contains lysine and rutin, which makes capillaries stronger and improves circulation, blood pressure and blood cholesterol.

Liquorice root is used in 50 per cent of all oriental and herbal medicines, because it contains glycyrrhizin and triterpenoids, which enhance immune functions, fight gum disease, gingivitis and tooth decay, and can improve liver function. It also has anti-tumour properties and guards against excessive oestrogens. It has proven very effective in the treatment of arthritis. Liquorice root is 50 times sweeter than sugar cane, yet it has no calories. You can make the root into a delicious tea. You can also buy liquorice tea. Sweet-shop liquorice has no benefits.

* Onions From the garlic family, onions have been used for centuries to ward off colds and other ailments. They are a recognised anti-cancer food because they are rich in quercetin – an antioxidant that inhibits cancer-causing agents. Onions are also anti-inflammatory, antibacterial, anti-fungal and antiviral, and they are also full of digestive enzymes. They have been proven to prevent cancer, particularly stomach cancer, and to cleanse and thin the blood. The quercetin protects against blood clotting. Onions are also full of allicin and glutathione, and they detoxify and boost the immune system. In Ireland, onions have been used for years to dissolve blood clots in horses. Red onions are by far the best, followed by yellow onions. White onions don't contain the same healing compounds or quercetin.

Olive oil is good for the heart, and people who regularly eat it also have less cancer, especially breast cancer, heart disease and lower levels of cholesterol. Olive oil is high in quercetin. It is a good fat that can reverse some of the oxidation damage caused by trans-fats. Oleocanthal, a compound in olive oil, has been found to slow down changes in the brain that lead to Alzheimer's. It is also anti-inflammatory and protects against heart disease.

Oats have been shown to reduce blood pressure and to reduce cholesterol levels by 3 per cent (or 7 per cent, if your cholesterol level is already high), just 55g (2oz) of oat bran daily can lower low-density lipoprotien (LDL) cholesterol (known as 'bad' cholesterol) by 15 per cent. Oats also contain phytoestrogens, which can prevent the harmful type of oestrogen from leading to breast cancer. Oatmeal rubbed onto the face or body and gently removed is a gentle natural and cheap exfoliant, far better for you than some of the cosmetic ones, which can contain harsh unnatural ingredients.

* **Parsley** Full of vitamins C and A, with some B vitamins, as well as iron, calcium and potassium, parsley is a natural diuretic and a great inner cleanser. Parsley is regarded in some circles and by some nutritionists as the third most powerful food on earth.

Peppers Red and yellow peppers are the best, being the highest in vitamin C. Peppers are high in glutathione, which is good for vision and neutralises bad fats. Glutathione is found only in fresh green, red and yellow vegetables; red peppers have more vitamin C than oranges.

* **Quinoa** is a seed used by the South American Incas. It is considered a super-food because it contains all eight essential amino acids and is very rich in calcium and iron, so it is a good replacement for meat or dairy produce. It is rather like rice, but cooks in half the time and is an energy-sustaining food eaten by many top athletes. It is great in soups, salads or casseroles.

* **Spinach** Full of antioxidants, spinach can help to deter strokes, cancer, heart disease and high blood pressure, among other things. Spinach deserves to be in the top ten of super-foods, because it contains lutein and zeaxanthin (which are claimed to be especially strong anti-ageing compounds and protect against macular eye degeneration) and folic acid, which offers protection to the brain and arteries, and is another anti-cancer agent. It also contains iron, calcium, potassium and more protein than any other vegetable. Like carrots, spinach is excellent at protecting the sight. It is also high in magnesium.

* **Seeds (sunflower, pumpkin, sesame, sprouted seeds)** Pumpkin and squash seeds are full of zinc, vitamins and minerals. Sunflower seeds are high in vitamin E and B vitamins. All seeds are high in magnesium and have some Omega-3 oils. They are also a good source of protein.

Thyme is a herb rather than a food, but I have included it because it has more anti-ageing compounds than any other herb, so it is worth adding thyme to your diet by including it in cooked dishes, salads, soups and making a herb tea from it.

* **Tomatoes** contain quercetin and the antioxidant lycopene, which is proven to be a super-efficient free-radical scavenger and preserves mental and physical functions in the elderly. Lycopene can also protect against cancer of the cervix, digestive tract, stomach, colon, prostate, lung and pancreas.[16] Eating ten servings of tomatoes every week can reduce the risk of prostate cancer in men by 35 per cent. Lycopene protects against age-related cell damage and oxidation. Lycopene is preserved during heating, so you can consume your intake of tomatoes raw, juiced and in sauces and cooked dishes.

Tumeric Curcumin, a substance in turmeric, can revitalise your skin because it interacts with collagen, the protein in the dermis, stabilising it, which boosts skin quality and helps reduce scarring.

Walnuts are a great source of copper. They can stop hair from turning grey and help it to retain its natural colour for longer.

Wheat germ is full of B vitamins, and wheat germ oil contains omega-3 oils. Wheat germ is a separate and different food from wheat, which is very adulterated.

* Yams and sweet potatoes Wild yams contain a precursor of the hormone progesterone. In some tribes, when women are going through the menopause they eat lots of yams and don't seem to suffer with hot flushes or depression. It is very useful to eat or juice yams, if you are menopausal. Japanese women equally seem to have little trouble with the menopause. This has been linked to the Japanese diet being rich in soya and Omega-3 fish oil. Sweet potatoes have more beta-carotene and vitamin C than other vegetables and are a rich source of DHEA, a hormone that helps the body defend itself against ageing.

Add to this list all orange and yellow fruits, such as peaches, melons, mangoes, papaya, pineapple, lemons, oranges and grapefruits; orange and yellow vegetables, such as squash, pumpkin, swedes and turnips; all deeply coloured fruits and vegetables such as watermelon (which contains lycopene) melon and aubergines.

The more dark green or richly red or yellow and orange the hue of fruits and vegetables, the richer the antioxidant content within them. Green leafy vegetables are also a good source of calcium and a good alternative to dairy produce and fish. They help to detoxify the body and boost the immune system. A study by Tufts University found that increasing the amount of vitamin C in your diet can reduce the risk of developing cataracts by 77 per cent. The National Cancer Institute label oranges a total package of every anti-cancer inhibitor in existence. Grapefruits contain compounds that lower blood cholesterol and may reverse atherosclerosis – which is the biggest killer of women over 60 in the West. Citrus fruits contain limones, which increase the manufacture of enzymes involved in detoxifying the body, and they also lower cholesterol and reduce plaque in the arteries. Grapefruits are an excellent source of glutathione; make sure you eat the pith as well, because many of the grapefruit's benefits are stored there. Grapefruits can't be taken with statins, ironically!

If you eat plenty of fruit and vegetables and include the listed super-foods in your diet, you will be getting plenty of fibre, which is also essential in any diet. Fibre can help fight heart disease, cancer, high cholesterol, blood pressure and atherosclerosis. Fibre is an indigestible substance that makes up a plant's structure. It passes through our digestive system without being broken down or digested and it takes cholesterol, bile acids and toxins out of our body during its journey. Most people are only aware of the importance of fibre in alleviating constipation, but it does much more than that. Cholesterol can build up in the blood and will lead to clogged arteries if it is not removed and passed out of the body as bile acids from the digestive tract. I am talking about plant fibre here, not bran or any grain fibre, which can be unhealthy.

Foods to avoid if you want to age well are:

- Cured meats, bacon, sausages and hot dogs, as they are very carcinogenic and full of harmful nitrates.
- Barbecued foods, because the smoke and heat of the barbecue may cause cancer compounds to form, particularly nitrosamine, the most powerful of all carcinogens. Don't barbecue too frequently; ensure the grill is high above the coals; and wrap the food, or even wrap the grill pan in foil to stop fat dripping onto the coals and causing even more smoke and heat.
- Hydrogenated fats, especially margarines and foods cooked in fat that may be rancid, such as crisps, popcorn, pre-packaged

foods, and so on. Hydrogenated oils increase the amount of free radicals in the body and cause damage to cells. They can also slow the supply of oxygen to the brain. Trans-fats, which are made by solidifying hydrogenated fats into margarine and shortening, need to be avoided because they cause so much cellular damage. The body simply can't get rid of them. They are banned in Demark and in some US states their use is restricted. One day they will be recognised as an incredibly cruel thing that man invented, and banned everywhere. They are found in cakes, biscuits, crisps and processed foods. One of the reasons Mediterranean countries have a lower incidence of heart disease is because they consume less bad fat and more good fat and they eat foods that are very high in quercetin, glutathione and lycopene. Safe and healthy fats are monounsaturated fats such as olive oil, fish oil, flaxseed oil, avocados, olives and almonds. Ensure you eat all the foods from the list that contain glutathione, because this helps to defuse free-radical activity from fats and can neutralise rancid fat.

- Artificial sweeteners – they are made from petrochemicals and are probably one of the unhealthiest substances that humans consume. Artificial sweeteners have been linked to Alzheimer's disease and to dementia and failing memory. You can take natural sweeteners such as stevia, xylitol and Zsweet, which are made from plants and are natural and safe.

- Foods that are high in sugar, heavily processed foods and foods full of preservatives and excessive salt.

Vital water

Water is an absolutely essential part of feeling and looking well. It is needed by every cell and tissue in the body. Water is essential for digestion and circulation and does everything from carrying nutrients throughout the body to taking waste and toxins out of the body. Our cells cannot regenerate or repair properly without water. If you are aiming for weight loss you need to drink enough water in order to be able to lose weight properly.

If you don't drink enough water, you won't be able to flush toxins out of your system. The toxins are then stored in fat so it is harder to lose weight. Also, without an adequate amount of water you're more likely to misinterpret thirst as hunger and overeat. The body needs a constant supply of water, because we lose so much every day through sweat and urine, and even through our breath. In order to look and feel younger, you must drink eight large glasses or 2 litres (3½ pints) of water daily. You need to drink it throughout the day, because if you try to take in a huge amount of water at one time your body will pass it out of your system again too quickly.

Because your body needs a constant supply of water, it is best to get into the habit of drinking a large glass on rising, then seven more throughout the day. Drinking enough water will be an asset to your skin and to your energy levels. Our bodies are made of 90 per cent water: our bones, blood cells, muscles and organs are all mostly composed of water. As we age, we lose more and more water from our bodies, causing our faces to look shrunken and our skin to look wrinkled.

Vitamins, supplements and ageing

Taking the right amount of vitamins and supplements has a very important part to play in looking, feeling and becoming years younger. Dr Linus Pauling, the renowned American scientist and twice winner of the Nobel Prize, believed that we could all add 16–24 years to our lives by eating a healthy balanced diet. He also believed that optimum nutrition was the medicine of the future.

Although it is true that the vitamins found in fruit and vegetables can be better than the vitamins taken in tablet form, we can no longer truly tell the vitamin content of the foods we buy and eat. The quality of the food we eat links directly to the quality of the soil it is grown in, and unfortunately much of our food is grown in soil that is very poor in minerals and selenium. Also, so much of our seemingly fresh food is irradiated and treated with pesticides and other agents that can counteract their vitamin benefits. A lot of food that we buy as fresh can be days, and sometimes weeks, old and its vitamin content will have been reduced by storage.

Organic produce is better because it is grown without pesticides and chemicals, but even some organic produce is grown in soil that is very poor and, again, lacking in selenium. Apart from growing your own food and regularly replenishing the soil, the only way you can be certain you are getting the vitamins essential for successful ageing is to take them in supplement form.

YOU'RE PROBABLY NOT GETTING ENOUGH

A survey conducted by the Ministry of Agriculture, Fisheries and Food reported that only one in ten people get even the basic recommended daily allowance (RDA) of nutrients from their food. Medical researcher Dr Stephen Davies tested the blood levels of vitamin B in thousands of people and found that seven out of ten were deficient. The RDA does not make allowances for people who smoke or drink, or who are recovering from illness or infection, or who live in a polluted city or are stressed or elderly, because the RDA is the recommended daily allowance for a person who is assumed to be already healthy.

If you have any problems with digestion and absorption, you may be passing vital elements straight out of your system (see the next section on digestion and ageing, page 237). A blood test can also show you the level of vitamins in your blood, so that you know how effective your absorption is, and it will show up any deficiencies you need to attend to.

Cooking can destroy most vitamins in food, including the allicin in garlic, which is a natural antibiotic. Even if you had the time and the tenacity to prepare fresh, organic and raw food daily you would have to eat masses of it to ensure your vitamin intake was sufficient to reverse ageing. Obviously this can be done, but it is time-consuming, it does not adapt well to eating out or accommodating the needs of family eating and some people don't digest raw food as well as food that is lightly cooked.

With some vitamins, such as vitamin E which is found in vegetable oils, fish oils, raw nuts, seeds and beans, you would need to eat a lot of oil and too many calories in order to get the amount of vitamins necessary.

If you think you are getting an abundance of vitamins in fruit juices, however, think again. Fresh juice is almost always pasteurised; juice made from concentrate has been heat-treated, so all the vitamins have been damaged. Juice is not a great food either because it's too high in sugar.

CHOOSING TO SUPPLEMENT

When supplementing vitamins it is essential to take the correct amount and to take all the vitamins that you need. Antioxidants work together; they are less effective on their own, but highly effective at detoxifying, fighting free radicals and slowing down age degeneration, and boosting the immune system when combined with other antioxidants and essential nutrients.

Vitamin supplements can strengthen the immune system and destroy newly formed cancer cells before they multiply, especially the vitamins A, C and E, the mineral selenium and beta-carotene. When taking vitamins to look and feel younger, it is important to remember that a lot of the effects are cumulative and retroactive. The vitamins are preventing signs of illness and ageing that you may not notice for 20 years. Below is a list of recommended vitamins, minerals or supplements, explaining the particular property of each. Although they are listed individually they do not need to be taken individually and many can be taken as a multivitamin mineral along with additional vitamins C and E and 1,000mg of fish oils.

Vitamins

Vitamin A helps to maintain young, smooth and soft skin, it reduces susceptibility to infection and can protect the lungs from pollution damage. It is essential for the maintenance of healthy skin, eyes, bones, hair and teeth. Take 10,000iu daily (iu means international units). Although 10,000iu sounds a lot it is a perfectly safe amount unless pregnant (if pregnant take no more than 7,500iu).

Vitamin B$_1$ helps to stimulate the immune system and is a natural antioxidant. It is also good for the digestion and nervous system.

Vitamin B$_2$ helps to prevent cataracts and to produce antibodies to fight infection. It is necessary for healthy skin and eyes and helps to release energy from foods.

Vitamin B$_3$ I recommend this to all my patients who are giving up smoking, because of its ability to promote blood flow and dilate the blood vessels damaged by smoking. This enables vital nutrients to be brought to the skin and helps cells detoxify. It is also excellent for digestion and for the nervous system and is essential for the maintenance of healthy skin and for proper mental functioning.

Vitamin B$_6$ helps to prevent arteriosclerosis – hardening of the arteries – and heart disease.

Vitamin B$_{12}$ helps to prevent anaemia and to maintain healthy red blood cells and a healthy nervous system. It boosts energy and can counteract depression. Take 500mcg. You can take all the B vitamins together as part of a multivitamin.

Vitamin C is essential for the manufacture of collagen. It helps to keep muscles firm and prevents skin from bagging, sagging and wrinkling as well as maintaining teeth, gums, bones and blood vessels. Vitamin C has been shown to reverse ageing by six years and is a superior free-radical scavenger and antioxidant. It helps to form red blood cells and can prevent internal bleeding and those hated and ageing broken veins. Vitamin C is also a natural healer, which is used in many cancer therapies. You can safely take up to 17g a day – some people take even more. A good guide is to take between 5 and 10g to slow down ageing (1g is 1,000mg). You can even increase the dose, since vitamin C is not stored in the body. You may find excess vitamin C has a laxative effect initially, so adjust the dose accordingly.

Vitamin D can slow down ageing while improving lifespan and quality of life. It can also help with psoriasis. Vitamin D is needed to help our bones absorb calcium. Without it they absorb only 10 per cent of calcium intake, but with it they absorb 80–90 per cent. It plays a key role in keeping bones and muscles strong. Take 800–1,000iu daily if you are over the age of 65. You should take vitamin D in the winter but don't need it in the summer, as long as your skin (preferably the skin on your arms) gets 20 minutes of sun daily.

Vitamin E has healing properties when applied to minor cuts, burns and abrasions. It is also super-nutrition for the skin and revitalising for when it is tired or stressed. Use pure, natural vitamin E in capsule form as a supplement to skin cream. Use it on cuts to prevent scarring and to prevent stretch marks. Free radicals are absorbed by vitamin E. It is effective in preventing and treating many diseases, including some cancers and heart disease, as well as offering resistance to many others. It boosts the immune system and repairs red blood cells. A *New England Journal of Medicine* study using over 87,000 women found that women who took vitamin E supplements for over two years had a 40 per cent lower risk of heart disease. It has also been proven to reduce sun damage to skin. Russian scientists using vitamin E on ageing patients found it increased stamina, strength and sleep patterns along with a disappearance of wrinkles, and even grey hair. You can safely take between 400 and 1,000iu daily.

Minerals

Beta-carotene offers great anti-ageing properties, and it protects the cells and tissues. It is excellent in protecting the skin, lungs and the immune system. Beta-carotene can also protect and treat the damaging effects of the sun's UV rays. Take 2,500iu or 6–30mg daily.

Calcium is vital for healthy teeth and bones and good for digestion. If you take a combined calcium–magnesium supplement, it can stop you craving sugar. If you are low in magnesium, you often have high blood pressure, can be prone to migraines and may crave sugar. Always take calcium supplements with meals, as the stomach acid produced while eating breaks down calcium carbonate and helps its absorption. Take 500–1,500mg daily.

Chromium has been shown to extend the lifespan in animals by 33 per cent. Take 100mg daily.

Selenium has anti-cancer properties. It offers protection from some types of cancer and heart problems and naturally detoxifies the body of metals and mercury. If you eat a lot of fish, take selenium. Selenium greatly improves immune function. It has been shown to reverse ageing and has been proven to reduce sun damage to the skin. The average daily intake of selenium is only 43mcg. The World Health Organization recommends between 50 and 200mcg as safe and adequate. Adults can safely take 300–400 mcg daily. All smokers and ex-smokers should take selenium, as it helps to block the growth of tumours.[17]

Sulphur Like chromium, sulphur has been shown to extend the lifespan of animals. It also protects the body from too much exposure to electricity. If you eat fish, meat and eggs on a weekly basis you shouldn't need to supplement sulphur – if you don't, take 2,500mg daily (in the form of MSM).

Zinc is another excellent antioxidant that fights free radicals. It is also good for improving memory and vision, maintaining fertility and libido, and improving the loss of taste or smell. Take 20–25mg daily.

Other supplements

Co-enzyme Q_{10} (CoQ_{10}) An excellent antioxidant that boosts immune function, CoQ_{10} has a protective effect on the heart and on cell membranes. It also converts energy from food to our cells and is recommended if you have poor digestion or absorption. Take 30mg daily.

Echinacea is a wonderful immune-system booster. It's a great thing to take as winter draws in because it boosts your immunity and can help prevent coughs and colds. It's also useful if you're about to fly because it can help you resist picking up infections on aeroplanes. Other times when it's useful are if you are under pressure, working late, or around sick people – or any time when you feel your immunity could be low.

Gamma linolenic acid (GLA) balances hormone function and is known to help with premenstrual syndrome (PMS) and the menopause. It also helps to keep joints supple and has a natural and proven anti-inflammatory effect. GLA is one of the essential fatty acids needed by our bodies to maintain the structure of cell membranes. In the body, GLA converts to a substance that regulates every cell and organ of the body and controls the activities of key enzymes. GLA has been shown to help dyslexic and hyperactive children, because a lack of essential fatty acids is indicated as a trigger for behavioural problems. It also protects against the effects of smoking and pollution and improves the skin. Take 2,000mg daily.

Ginkgo biloba is a powerful antioxidant, which seems to have an anti-ageing effect on the brain. It can reverse a declining memory and is excellent at improving blood circulation, especially to the brain and scalp, so this is recommended if you have thinning hair. *Ginkgo biloba* carries oxygen and blood to diseased areas of the body and is known as a 'smart drug' because of its ability to improve and restore memory, concentration and circulation. *Ginkgo biloba* also contains bioflavonoids. Take 80mg daily.[18]

Japanese green tea is a powerful antioxidant and metabolism booster. It contains chemicals called methylxanthines, which seem to boost metabolism, helping to burn fat more rapidly. It also reduces cholesterol. It can be bought as the leaf or in teabags and even comes in capsule form from health-food shops.

Spirulina is a freshwater-growing alga which is a natural antioxidant that can improve skin texture. Algae are one of the phenomena in nature that never grow old. Spirulina contains concentrated amounts of all the nutrients found in green vegetables. It was used in Minsk on all children suffering from radiation poisoning after Chernobyl, because spirulina was able to help detoxify their bodies. Only buy the best kind of spirulina, which has been grown under controlled conditions. Doses will vary according to whether you buy it in powder or tablet form; you will need about 16 tablets or 3 large spoonfuls daily.

Choose the supplements from the above list to suit your age and state of health. Everyone should take a multivitamin–mineral, plus selenium, omega-3 oils and CoQ_{10}. Add *Ginkgo biloba* if you are over 50 and have a poor memory or hair loss. Take any other supplement listed above that relates to your particular situation.

Digestion and ageing

Good digestion is linked to ageing well, whereas poor digestion can accelerate the ageing process and disrupt every system in the body, including cell regeneration. If you have digestion problems, food is not absorbed properly into the blood or assimilated into cells and tissues, leaving you nutritionally deficient regardless of how good your diet is.

Digestion is essential to good health and to looking and remaining young. If our digestion is functioning at less than 100 per cent, it follows that we are also less than 100 per cent. If you have inadequate digestion, taking all the foods and vitamins listed previously won't have a positive effect on your body, because they will not be fully absorbed. Some people have digestion that is so bad that they don't even absorb 10 per cent of the vitamins or nutrients in their diet.

Digestion is a complex process, using acids, alkalis and enzymes. Digestion uses up huge amounts of energy, which is why when we overeat we tend to feel sleepy or we fall asleep. This is because the brain diverts oxygen and blood away from major organs in order to use it in digestion. Many people have digestion problems. Disorders of the stomach, intestines, gall bladder, liver and pancreas can all lead to poor digestion, as does existing or having existed on a diet of over-processed and over-refined food. Eating food full of preservatives means that the same preservative that stopped bacteria growing on your potato or piece of bread will also stop your digestive system from being able to work fully. When faced with preservatives, the body has to make more and more digestive juices in order to break down food, and then it becomes so overworked it eventually works less efficiently. This is another reason for buying more organic produce.

HELP FROM DIGESTIVE ENZYMES

Tension can disrupt digestion, because eating when tense, tired, emotional or overwrought will interfere with the free flow of digestive enzymes, leaving the eater with indigestion and very little or no energy released from the food. Just a look at the sales figures for indigestion pills and antacids is proof enough of the enormous number of people with digestion problems. In England, over 67 million are sold yearly; however, many people don't understand the long-term effects that poor digestion has on general health and on ageing.

If you are suffering from poor digestion, wonderful help is at hand in the form of digestive enzymes, which help to digest food when your own digestive system fails to complete the process.

There are many enzymes involved in digestion, including pepsin, trypsin, rennin and pancreatin. By taking digestive enzymes you are helping your body to absorb food and get all the vitamins it needs, and you are maintaining improved energy, because when you don't digest food properly your body is forced to take blood from your brain and muscles in an attempt to re-digest food, leaving you feeling sleepy and lacking energy.

When we don't digest food correctly, it tends to sit in the stomach while the body makes more attempts at digestion. Eventually, the food will ferment and putrefy, producing toxic elements, which cause the skin to break out and look sallow. This process also causes a host of other unpleasant effects, which include premature ageing, allergies, headaches, lethargy, depression and being more prone to protruding veins. These all result from our body being forced to re-absorb poisons.

Taking digestive enzymes can eliminate all these symptoms. If your digestion is poor, I recommend you take them with every meal. If you have poor digestion only when you overeat or eat certain types of food, take them then, and always keep some digestive enzymes in your purse or wallet – they are miracle workers. I don't take them all the time, but I always have some to hand, I usually find myself giving them away to people who might benefit from them – and they always do.

PROBLEMS WITH STOMACH ACID

Studies have shown that up to 40 per cent of the elderly may have hypochlorhydria, a condition in which the stomach is not acid enough, leading to mineral deficiencies arising from poor digestion, which can in turn lead to osteoporosis and fragile bones. Taking calcium supplements won't always help, because people with hypochlorhydria can't absorb calcium or magnesium carbonate.

DO YOU HAVE DIGESTION PROBLEMS?

I had poor digestion for years before I understood its far-reaching effects. Like many people, I was concerned only with treating the symptoms rather than tackling the cause.

It's quite easy to establish whether or not you have digestion problems by answering these few simple questions:

After eating, do you:

- Feel bloated or swollen; do you need to loosen clothing or does clothing feel uncomfortably tight for long periods?
- Get a lot of gas?
- Feel nausea or have stomach pain?
- Feel tired, sleepy or lethargic?
- Get headaches?
- Sometimes get diarrhoea? Or constipation?

If you are experiencing any of these symptoms, you have poor digestion or malabsorption. This means that you aren't absorbing or benefiting from the nutrients in your food. It also means that your body is working too hard at digestion. When this happens frequently, the body is forced to leech enzymes out of other organs, such as the pancreas, to use for digestion.

The enzymes used in digestion are also used in cell renewal and have a vital part to play in preventing disease and age degeneration. We must have a sufficient supply of pancreatic enzymes in order for cells to work properly and in order to sustain immunity to many illnesses such as cancer. When enzymes are continually being removed from the pancreas for digestion it has a dreadful effect on ageing.

The same thing happens if you always eat very late at night and then go to bed. First, you won't enjoy proper sleep, because your body is busy digesting food instead of resting. Second, your body takes enzymes from the pancreas to digest the food when these enzymes are already earmarked to be used in the process of cellular repair, renewal and rebuilding of the body, which always takes place at night, and also to fight any developing cancer. If your body is digesting, the whole process of cell repair and regeneration is set aside and, although this is acceptable occasionally, it has a terrible effect on your health and appearance if it is happening too frequently.

TIPS FOR EATING TO BENEFIT YOUR DIGESTION

I'm not a killjoy – I wouldn't dream of suggesting you cease going out to dinner or having late-night dinner parties, especially since this is something I enjoy myself. Here are the changes you can make that will allow you to enjoy yourself while maintaining optimum health and looking young:

- Don't regularly eat very late at night. If you like to eat something late, eat fruit, because it is raw and it is easily and quickly digested. Also, your metabolic rate is at its lowest in the evening, so if you starve all day and then eat late at night, you will find it much harder to lose weight if you are overweight.

- Always take digestive enzymes when you do eat at night. They will do the job of breaking down and digesting the food for you, leaving your pancreas free to do its perfect work repairing cells.
- Eat less cooked food at night, and more raw. Include foods like pineapple and papaya, which are full of natural digestive enzymes. Cooked food tends to be food without enzymes. Raw foods of plant and vegetable origin retain enzymes when eaten and thus don't need to take enzymes from the body for use in digestion.
- Don't eat when you are feeling very stressed or very tired or emotional, because tension will limit the free flow of digestive enzymes. If you feel you have to eat and you are feeling very tense or tired, take digestive enzymes.
- Don't eat too quickly. Slow down and chew your food. Much digestion begins in the mouth, but when you rush your food your body is unable to absorb the nutrients contained in it. Don't eat too much.
- Don't eat too many varieties of food at each meal because this makes it much harder for the body to digest. Also avoid very rich or spicy food – the more simple and basic your food is the easier it is to digest.
- Refined food and dairy are very hard to digest. A good rule of thumb is that the body is designed to digest food that grows or roams on the earth and in the trees – natural foods that are lightly cooked. Cheese and milk don't come into this category, because they are so concentrated and were never designed for human consumption – don't eat a lot of dairy produce.

Ice cream and cheese are notoriously hard to digest. It is said that some 80 per cent of the world's population cannot digest milk protein properly. This is known as lactose intolerance, or an inability to digest dairy produce. Children under ten are more easily able to digest milk products, because they have an enzyme in their bodies called lactase, which is specifically there to digest lactose. Without lactase, an enzyme that declines in humans from age ten, most dairy produce will go through the digestive system undigested.

To make matters worse, dairy produce contains casein, which is an insoluble protein that plugs up the intestinal tract. Cooked cheese, especially, sticks to the walls of the intestines like glue. Yoghurt is easier to digest, because of the healthy bacteria it contains – the live, active cultures in real yoghurt break down lactose in the intestines, so natural live yoghurt is an exception to the rule on dairy.

Wheat is another product that many people have problems digesting, because it is so over-processed and usually grown with an abundance of chemicals and pesticides. People eat wheat too often – for breakfast, lunch and dinner in the form of bread, cereals, cakes, biscuits, pies, sandwiches, pizza, pasta, noodles, crackers, snack bars and a variety of other foods – building up intolerance. Until we had mills, no one ate large quantities of wheat. It is a modern, unhealthy food. White flour mixed with water makes great glue – the gluten in flour, and flour products, when eaten as part of a food such as bread, becomes a glue-like substance that sticks to the intestinal wall and to other foods passing through the intestine. It does not pass out of the body very easily and can remain in the intestines for years. If you have gluten intolerance you should know that there is not an organ in the body that is not affected by gluten.

WHO SHOULD TAKE DIGESTIVE ENZYMES?

Even if you feel your digestion is good, it is still worth taking digestive enzymes every time you have a heavy meal, a late meal or a meal that is greatly varied or based on over-processed food. Many people who are serious about wanting to look younger and feel great take digestive enzymes daily as a matter of course.

If you seem to be intolerant to some foods but you can't resist the occasional pizza or ice cream, take digestive enzymes to minimise the damage, but don't use them as an excuse to eat a terrible diet. Even if you take digestive enzymes with every meal, you still need to pay attention to your diet and eat more natural, healthy and, preferably, organic food and less processed, refined and junk food.

WHICH ENZYMES SHOULD YOU CHOOSE?

The best type of digestive enzymes are vegetable based – papaya digestive enzymes are good. Chlorella, from the spirulina family, is a natural digestive enzyme. You can buy digestive enzymes in any health-food shop. My favourites are made by Solgar and Higher Nature.

Electricity and ageing

The effects of electricity on our bodies is something that has only recently been realised since only a few generations ago people had very little electricity in their homes, just the lights and a radio. Even in the last 15 years our use of personal electric items has massively increased, with the advent of mobile phones, smartphones, laptop computers, electronic games, tablet computers and the like.

When I bought my first home about 30 years ago it was a new conversion and yet it had only two socket points in the bedroom and three in the lounge. This was normal and sufficient.

When I converted my new home nine years later, I had to have two twin sockets on every wall, and even more in the living room, because, like many householders, I had then acquired a computer, a printer, a cordless phone, a mobile phone, an answering machine, a CD and DVD player, a shredder, a wifi and a satellite system.

In my kitchen I had a microwave, a juicer, a blender, a steamer and slow cooker – all competing for power sockets. Sometimes I think of the home my grandmother had only 35 years ago and how she would have been so baffled by all our gadgets.

Worst of all, I noticed I was sleeping under two bedside electric lights with my answering machine, my cordless phone and mobile phone and alarm clock all plugged in and sitting on my bedside table.

LIMIT ELECTRICITY WHERE YOU SLEEP

If you want to look and feel younger, you must limit the amount of electricity that is around you as you sleep. It also helps to be aware of the electricity you are close to during the day. Night-time exposure to electricity, however, is even more important, because we stay in one place for several hours, so all the electricity by our beds, especially that near to our pillows, is passing in and out of our bodies and our cells all night long. This disrupts cell activity at the time when cells are programmed to do the very important work of cell regeneration and repair, which is essential to our looks and health.

While I was studying the effects of electricity on the body, I made some very easy changes. I put my CD player on the floor, further away from me but near enough that I can listen to it. Phones, laptop and iPads are all charged downstairs, and if I need my mobile nearby at night, I leave it outside the bedroom door. I got rid of my alarm clock; however, if you feel one is essential, get a very small battery-operated model, *not* a fluorescent one. I have a normal handset phone by the bed, not an electric cordless one. I moved my answering machine downstairs, and although I do occasionally love to watch television in bed I have moved my TV right to the end of my room, as we must keep electrical appliances 2.1m (7ft) away from us to screen the electromagnetic rays that come from them.

LIVING IN A MODERN ELECTRIC AGE BUT WITH UNCHANGED BIOLOGY

We have moved so quickly into a world where we are bombarded by, and seemingly always in the company of, something electric, yet we don't fully know the effects of, say, using a mobile phone for hours at a time. They don't come with any warning, but they do have a detrimental effect on our body cells, as does spending too long in too close proximity to any electrical appliance. We are in contact day and night with electromagnetic rays, and the effects of electrical pollution are beginning to be linked to many illnesses and ailments, including low sperm count, infertility, myalgic encephalitis (ME), migraines, cancer, depression and attention deficit hyperactivity disorder (ADHD), to name just a few.

Scientists and doctors are now becoming increasingly aware of the negative debilitating effects that too much, or too frequent, exposure to household electricity can have on the body. In most modern homes, without us being aware of it, electromagnetic rays are passing through our delicate body cells day and night – often 24 hours a day. Our bodies are not designed to cope with this, and it has happened far too fast for the human body to adapt to electrical pollution. You can feel the electricity if you run your hand over the television screen; just switching on a lamp will instantly cause the brain's rhythms to change; and if you were to hold a strip light near to an electricity pylon it could come on just because of the electricity that is present.

People whose homes are close to electric sub-stations, power lines or pylons do seem to have a higher incidence of illnesses, including some forms of cancer, Alzheimer's and Parkinson's disease, as well as depression, insomnia and lethargy.

The same thing can occur in homes that have an abundance of electrical equipment in almost every room.

AVOID RADIATION AND ELECTROMAGNETIC FIELDS

X-rays are also a concern. Many people just don't want to believe this, but it has finally been accepted and proven that over-exposure to X-ray machines can cause cancer and other illnesses. Ross Adey, chairman of the US National Council on Radiation Protection, states that there is proof that even very low levels of exposure to electromagnetic fields (EMFs) is linked to long-term effects on health.

The report suggests limiting our exposure to a maximum of 0.2 microteslas – the measurement of leakage. In most homes the levels measure about 0.1–0.2; however, the closer you are to an appliance, the higher the level is. Being too close to the television or radio – and even being too close to a hairdryer – can immediately push the level up to 7.0. Many ordinary household appliances can emit a hundred times the limit recognised as safe, as soon as we are within 30cm (12in) of them, so the further away we are, the safer the limit becomes: even with something as simple as vacuuming you can benefit your health by keeping the vacuum at arm's length rather than holding it right next to your body.

Electromagnetic fields are measured in nanoteslas. The safe level, according to leading American and Swedish reports, is 200 nanoteslas. To keep to this safe level you need to sleep at least 1.2m (4ft) away from electricity meters, clock radios and electrical appliances, or the level can go up enormously. I realise this sounds alarming, but the good news is that these same levels go down significantly as you move further away from the electricity. Moving 30cm (12in) away makes a huge difference and is easy to do. Don't keep your mobile phone in your pocket all day or have it right next to you while watching television at night. If you are in front of a computer screen all day, use a shield to protect you from the rays.

THE IMPORTANCE OF JUST BEING AWARE

I am not suggesting that we give up our electrical devices, but that we become aware of their negative side effects. Don't let children sleep with a computer or television by the bed – move appliances as far away from the bedhead as possible, preferably outside the bedroom. Even when appliances are turned off they still emit a frequency so charge them outside the bedroom.

Put stereos, radios and alarm clocks on the floor, especially if there are very small children in the room.

The effects of electromagnetic rays passing through the body constantly during the night are very detrimental to looking and feeling young. To look young and to have good skin and good health we need to have strong resilient cells – we must protect our cells from electrical pollution, especially at night, since this is when cells regenerate and repair.

QUICK TIPS FOR REDUCING ELECTRICITY EXPOSURE

Here are some very easy changes that you can make to benefit your health and remain younger:

- Don't fall asleep watching television in bed.
- Watch television from a distance of about 1m (3ft) preferably 1.2m (4ft).
- Move as many surplus electric appliances out of your bedroom as you can.
- Place those you feel that you must keep as far away from your bed as possible.

- If you feel you must have a bedside clock, have a tiny battery one.
- Downsize your bedside light – push it further away from your pillows. Aim to sleep 1.2m (4ft) away from electricity, even if it means you have to push lamps away from your pillows at night.
- Sleep at least 1.2m (4ft) away from storage heaters, electricity meters, clock radios and electrical sockets too, if you can.
- Don't sit or stand too close to electrical appliances.
- Don't sleep with your head near a radiator.
- Don't use an electric blanket, especially an electric over-blanket designed to be left switched on all night.
- Remember your hairdresser's advice: keep the dryer more than 35cm (14in) away from your head. This advice is given to protect your hair from burning, but it will protect your body too.
- Take high doses of vitamin C, at least 1,000mg daily, as it offers protection against radiation – as does sulphur and spirulina. Take at least 10 capsules of spirulina daily; treble that amount if you work close to electrical appliances. Foods rich in sulphur are broccoli, Brussels sprouts, cabbage, cauliflower and eggs.
- Cut down your use of appliances, and when you do use them, use them for less time.
- Replace your cordless phone with a normal handset phone.
- Be aware of how long you are talking on a mobile phone. Don't use it when you can use a regular phone. The same applies to cordless phones: use a normal handset phone whenever possible, as both mobile phones and cordless phones are very highly charged. When you are using a mobile phone, keep changing sides, as you hold it to you; don't clamp the phone to your ear or mouth, hold it a little way away and don't stay on the phone for too long. Note that using an earpiece with a mobile phone may not stop you having the phone too close to you.

- Use a protective screen if you use a computer, and take frequent breaks – perhaps go outside away from electricity for a few minutes every few hours. Spider plants and cacti are apparently good at absorbing radiation from computer terminals, so place one behind your computer. I placed a spider plant behind my computer: it has grown enormous so it must like it. Rose quartz crystal is also good at absorbing radiation.
- Notice how much you are around electricity and make changes that are appropriate and effective for you, your health and your looks.
- With small children, make some decisions to restrict their exposure to electricity. Encourage children to sit further away from the television.

I love my gadgets and would not want to give up my laptop, my iPhone or my TV, but I have made very many changes that have not inconvenienced me at all, and I urge you to do the same.

Exercise and ageing

'A feeble body enfeebles the mind'

Jean-Jacques Rousseau (1712–78)

If you want to become and remain younger, it is vital to engage in some form of regular exercise, because exercising has a very important role to play in slowing down ageing. In numerous tests exercising has been proven, beyond all doubt, to prevent muscle wastage and bone loss while maintaining agility and boosting energy levels. Regular and gentle exercise alone will reverse ageing by five years in men and four in women, according to scientist Dr Richard Hochschild, while regular aerobic exercise can cause the heart to be biologically ten years younger. Studies by Harvard and Stanford universities involving 17,000 men and women carried out over 50 years found exercise unquestionably delays ageing.

Tufts University ran an eight-week strength-training programme, taking the oldest and frailest people in an old people's home and involving them in a gentle programme of weight-bearing exercises. The results found that women and men between the ages of 87 and 96 could increase their muscle size and strength by 300 per cent within just eight weeks while also improving co-ordination and balance. Tests carried out at the Andrus Gerontology Center in California took over 200 inactive 60 and 70 year olds and placed them on a programme of moderate exercise. They found that they became as fit as people 30 years younger, with energy levels to match.

In another study, people between the ages of 80 and 90 years who did gentle and regular exercise doubled their strength. Even gentle exercise will reverse ageing by 10 per cent. Swimming, walking, yoga and t'ai chi are all excellent, because they are easy to do and don't put any strain on the body. Exercise can reverse ten major effects of ageing, such as high blood pressure, increased body fat, decreased muscle mass, reduced hearing and reduced bone density. Exercise strengthens heart muscles making the heart pump more efficiently.

It can even improve hearing and memory. Exercise helps constipation greatly, because it improves bowel transit time by up to 56 per cent. It has a positive effect on motilin, a gastro-intestinal hormone linked to faster transit time of waste through the bowel. Exercise also improves blood flow to the intestines, improving bowel movements in a safe and comfortable way. Constipation is itself very ageing, because toxins that should be eliminated are absorbed by the bowel and transferred back into the bloodstream. The result is that we can get headaches, we feel sluggish, our skin looks grey and unhealthy, and we can break out in spots. Constipation can also cause varicose veins.

You don't need to overdo exercise or strain your body to get excellent results. Gentle exercise is just as effective. Bengt Saltin, a Swedish physiologist, ran some tests in the 1960s where five men, two of whom were athletes, were asked to lie in bed for three weeks while he monitored their bodies' physiological responses to extended disuse. His results showed that within just 21 days their aerobic capacity diminished so much that it was equivalent to 20 years of ageing. When they began to exercise again they were able to reverse the results within a few weeks – proof that exercise reverses ageing.

THE DANGERS OF INACTIVITY

If you stay inactive for 24 hours, your muscle tissue starts to decline; if you have to endure even short periods of bed rest your bones quickly lose minerals and become weaker and more prone to breaking; your muscles shrink and you begin to experience skin and muscle wasting. The major cause of muscle loss as we age is being inactive. Inactivity is an enemy of ageing. If you plan to become and remain younger, you must take part in some form of regular exercise. We can improve our bodies by using them more, not less.

In tribes and cultures where daily exercise is the norm, osteoporosis and osteoarthritis are virtually unknown. It has been proven again and again that we cannot wear out our bodies by using them the way they were meant to be used, which is by being active. Although it is true that excessive exercise can have a detrimental effect on joints, what I am talking about here is gentle, easy and regular exercise that can be enjoyed at any age. Deepak Chopra, a leading authority on ageing, has said, 'We don't wear out, and too much rest can be the worst thing for our body and for muscle and skeletal wasting.'

Not exercising is harder work than exercising. Dr De Vries at the Gerontology Center in California said, 'It is the body so unused to activity that tires at the slightest effort.' The great thing about exercise is that once you begin to exercise you start to enjoy it and want to continue. It is never ever too late to begin an exercise programme, as the Tufts University programme shows, even beginning exercising at 90 will benefit your body. But don't wait, start to exercise now and you will benefit in many ways.

DON'T LET BAD SCHOOL EXPERIENCES TURN YOU OFF

When I was at school I hated all forms of exercise and sports and was definitely unsporty and classed as no good at sport. I left school believing that I hated exercise and was hopeless at it. I didn't exercise at all for several years, and I regret now that I was not athletic and missed out on all the pleasures of sport. Many years later, because I was studying physiology and because my boyfriend was a professional footballer, I almost by accident became involved in the exercise boom, and after training I became an exercise instructor. I found that I loved exercising and was very good at it and very good at teaching it. I found I was naturally supple. I could do the splits with ease and had lots of stamina; people in my class found it hard to believe I had not always been that way and had in fact only been exercising for a relatively short period of time. I taught classes in London, Los Angeles, Chicago, Washington DC and New York and appeared on *Newsnight*, and other television programmes, discussing the merits of exercise. I received a lot of very positive comments in articles in the press for my teaching; one said that I was the most professional and thorough exercise teacher in London. I often wondered how my schoolteachers felt about that, since they had told me repeatedly that I was hopeless at sport.

No matter what you have believed about yourself and exercising, it is never too late to begin and, like me, you might just surprise yourself and find that you love it, especially if you make a point of finding some kind of exercise that you enjoy in an environment that you like.

It's important to find a form of exercise that you really like so that you will stick with it. If you participate in any form of exercise and dislike it you won't reap beneficial results. It also helps to vary your exercise, so you could swim or walk, practise yoga and do some weight-bearing exercise every week. Sex is a very good exercise too.

WHAT SHOULD YOU DO AND HOW OFTEN?

It is just as effective to exercise little and often, and if you can find something like badminton or tennis that is social and enjoyable that's even better, as you will have more chance of sticking to it.

Whatever form of exercise you choose to do, you must include weight-bearing exercise in your programme, because weight-bearing exercise prevents thinning of the bones that results in osteoporosis. Bones are full of blood vessels and are constantly making new cells. Exercise that puts weight on the bones is essential to prevent bone loss. Lack of exercise is indicated as one of the causes of bone loss. It is important to begin an easy weight-bearing routine before you actually need to and to make it a way of life. Bone loss ultimately leads to lack of exercise so don't put it off – make exercise a part of your life.

It was found that astronauts who had spent weeks in space in a weightless state, which therefore put no weight on their bones, suffered dramatic bone loss that was remedied only by doing weight-bearing exercises. Astronauts have also become extremely prone to depression when their bodies have been forced to be inactive because of weightlessness.

Walter Bortz, a specialist in ageing at Stanford University, studied what happens to the body when we stop exercising and found that when the body is removed from physical exercise this alone will accelerate the ageing process. Our bodies need to exercise and like to be used. When we stop exercising a number of things happen: the heart becomes weaker; the arteries become older; the cardiovascular system becomes poorer; the muscle, skeletal and bone-wasting begins a rapid onset; bones become fragile and osteoporosis becomes a bigger risk; depression and weight gain become more apparent; and the body ages biologically so that it is older than its chronological years. When we stop using our bodies, they begin to fade and wither away. Dr Bortz called this 'disuse syndrome': a syndrome when the body stops exercising and begins to rapidly and prematurely age.

Dr Bortz has shown time and time again that lack of exercise produces changes in the body that parallel the changes we experience with ageing. He believes that some instances of rapid ageing are not symptoms of ageing at all, but symptoms of disuse of the body, because of failure to use it through exercise. His tests carried out on ageing people showed that exercise would reverse their symptoms and prevent them reoccurring for many years.

Dr Bortz said, 'So exceptional is the ability of regular exercise to reverse ageing, it seems extremely unlikely that any further drug or physician-oriented technique will approach such a benefit.'

EXERCISE STRENGTHENS THE BONES

By taking up regular weight-bearing exercise, you will increase the stress on your bones and this helps to increase bone density that in turn strengthens the bones. Women gradually lose bone mass from age 35 onwards. This increases more rapidly after menopause and bones become more brittle with the decrease of oestrogen. Putting weight on the bones through weight-bearing exercises can counteract much of this loss of bone mass.

Weight training is also known as strength training. You don't have to become a weight lifter to benefit from weight-bearing exercises, because using your own body as the weight is also an excellent form of weight training. You can find a programme in your local gym involving the use of small hand weights or appropriate weight-training machines. Many exercise classes use small hand weights as part of the class. If the idea of going to a gym does not appeal to you, you can do weight-bearing exercises at home utilising your body weight as resistance. Doing press-ups, or standing press-ups against a wall, is a way of using your own body weight, as are stomach exercises and leg and arm exercises using your own body weight as resistance.

Even walking is a weight-bearing exercise, because you are using a combination of gravity and your body weight on your legs and bones, which become stronger as more weight is brought to bear upon them. Walking also exercises your heart and lungs while toning muscles and burning calories. Walking for 30 minutes five or six times a week is as effective in slowing down and reversing ageing as running 40 miles a week. You don't have to work out hard, or push yourself or drip sweat to get the benefits that will allow you to defy ageing. Doing weight-bearing exercises three times a week will lower your risk of osteoporosis, as will two hours of walking every week. If your excuse has been, 'I don't have time to exercise', you need to know that 10 minutes of running or jogging a day will give you exactly the same benefits but you will need to run four or five days out of seven.

THE ALL-ROUND BENEFITS OF WEIGHT TRAINING

Weight training or strength training will also improve your posture, your body shape and your strength while it improves the density of bones that decrease with age. When muscle mass and strength diminish we become weaker, muscle is then replaced by fat, but if you participate in strength training you can maintain muscle tissue as you age, which will also keep you leaner with a better metabolism too, because muscle tissue is more metabolically active than fat tissue. The University of Pittsburgh School of Medicine studied 500 women for three years, recording their weight, triglycerides, cholesterol and blood pressure, at the beginning and at the end of the three-year period, and found that the women who exercised gained the least weight and had the healthiest blood cholesterol levels. The results of these tests, and those undertaken by other institutes set up to study the connection between exercise and ageing, show that exercise strengthens bones, prevents osteoporosis and weight increase while improving triglycerides, cholesterol and diastolic blood pressure.

These studies also show that exercise can decrease cholesterol levels while increasing metabolic rate, bone strength and memory, especially short-term memory. As we get older our brain cells may receive less nutrients and oxygen, but regular exercise can maintain high nutrient and oxygen levels which, in turn, fight ageing. Exercise also boosts endorphin levels and can decrease premenstrual syndrome (PMS).

From birth we make a hormone called human growth hormone (HGH). This hormone does very important work in the body. Primarily it increases muscle tone and lean mass while stimulating tissue growth and the growth of bones and organs. HGH is also responsible for enhancing the body's flexibility, thickening our muscles and maintaining healthy body tissues. HGH is naturally released into our bloodstream during the night, but it begins to decline at around the age of 30 and continues to drop until, by the age of 60, a third of men have either very little or no HGH; women at 60 still have some but not enough. After each session of intense exercise or a workout, however, we receive a dose of HGH.

You need HGH to remain young, but it naturally declines after the age of 30; however, you have it within your power to continue to receive a steady supply of HGH by exercising regularly. It must be a form of exercise that makes you work (but it does not have to be excessively hard work) and weight training, again, comes into this category perfectly.

In tests carried out in the US in 1989, 28 men, aged between 60 and 80, were given weekly injections of HGH. They very quickly reversed the age of their bodies by 20 years.

More studies from Florida show that 60-year-olds who had not exercised for years and had no muscle tone for 15 years, once put on to a weight-training programme, could gain muscle mass equal to that of someone of 21 and, as a bonus, their energy levels could match someone in their early twenties.

This is all the proof you need that exercise can, and does, fight ageing. You can be as strong and as fit in your seventies and eighties as you were in your twenties, with a consistent supply of HGH contributing to good muscle tone and flexibility, and continuing to build bones, organs and healthy body tissue no matter what your age.

THE EFFECTS OF ALCOHOL ON GROWTH HORMONES

One of the reasons alcohol is so ageing is because while you are drinking alcohol you will temporarily suppress the production of growth hormones, which keep your cells vigorous and active. Drinking alcohol too frequently may have a very detrimental effect on the production of growth hormones, as blood levels of growth hormones fall after every drinking bout. Heavy drinking also causes a dramatic increase of free radicals in our bodies and is very damaging to the skin. It can lead to blotchiness, broken veins, enlarged pores, puffiness, decreased skin tone, thin, stressed and tired skin and rhinophyma – a condition that causes the nose to become larger and redder. Alcohol can also disrupt menstrual periods and contribute to an early menopause. Alcohol can increase oestrogen levels by 20–30 per cent during mid-cycle. Alcohol dramatically ages the skin and lowers our bone mass, which can lead to osteoporosis. As we age, our bodies are less and less able to deal with alcohol.

If you are living a life of constant stress, or if you feel stressed all the time, you are undoubtedly affecting your ageing process and accelerating it. This is because 90 per cent of our cells' energy is needed for cell renewal, and in times of stress the whole process of rebuilding is set aside. This is OK if it happens only occasionally, but in the long term it has an appalling effect on our bodies and can age us far too quickly. There are so many methods available that counteract stress: for example, you can use massage, relaxation techniques and meditation to counteract stress; you can also learn deep breathing, which helps greatly; you can make a point of listening to any of the downloads that come with this programme when you feel stressed, and you will find them deeply relaxing; and taking regular exercise, such as swimming, yoga or walking, is a great stress reducer and yet another reason for taking regular exercise.

If you find a form of exercise that you love and that you find exciting or thrilling – or even adventurous – you will begin to age wonderfully, because excitement, thrills and adventure release very different chemicals in our brain and increase the flow of blood and oxygen to our body tissues. You don't need to go rock climbing to feel excitement; many people find that going to aerobics, or low-impact pilates or yoga classes, makes them feel so good that they find exercising compelling and fit it into their schedule as a priority, even finding classes to take while on holiday. Deep diaphragmatic breathing, which happens as you exercise, delivers more oxygen to the cells to activate cellular metabolism and helps toxins to leave the body.

Care for your feet

Our feet shorten as we age. The arch of the foot collapses, and many older people shuffle instead of walking. There is a specific exercise that will lengthen the foot arch – it is very easy to do.

Exercise 16: Strengthen the foot arches

1 To keep the arch of the foot in good condition, kneel on a mat or carpet without shoes and with your bottom resting on your heels and your palms or fingers placed on the floor either side of your knees.

2 Keeping your body weight distributed between your bottom and hands, and with your back reasonably straight, lift both your knees together off the floor and hold that position. The higher you can raise your knees, the more of a stretch you will feel in the arch of your foot.

3 Do this several times and hold for about 20 seconds.

4 You can get just as good results if you kneel but have your arms out ahead of you holding on to a chair or table for extra support.

Skin brushing and ageing

'To win back my youth ... there is nothing I wouldn't do except take exercise, get up early or be a useful member of the community'

Oscar Wilde (1854–1900)

Dry skin brushing, in sweeping upward movements, stimulates your lymph and blood circulation and removes impurities. It has the most amazing benefits: after just a few days of skin brushing you will find that you have masses more energy and your whole system will feel clean and invigorated, while your skin will already look and feel better and younger. The technique of skin brushing has been practised in Europe for centuries, especially at spas where it is used to stimulate lymphatic drainage and improve waste elimination via the skin's surface. It is often a very important part of natural healing and remedies.

Lymphatic drainage, correctly and professionally used, has been an effective treatment for some illnesses as well as fatigue and lethargy. It is also used as a beauty and anti-ageing treatment. Skin brushing stimulates circulation and helps pump blood down through the veins and up through the arteries, feeding the organs. It stimulates and cleanses the lymphatic system and promotes super-efficient lymphatic drainage while boosting the nervous system and improving the metabolic system. When you skin brush over the major lymph glands – which are situated in the armpits, groin, behind the elbows and knees, and either side of the throat, where waste fluid is deposited – it will stimulate the elimination of cellulite.

THE CAUSES OF CELLULITE

Cellulite is caused by impacted lymph and other waste material, along with fat, water and toxins, becoming trapped in areas of the body – usually the bottom and legs – and it is held by toughened connective tissue. If you are serious about wanting to be free of cellulite, then skin brush twice daily to stimulate the tissues beneath the skin, but not just before sleeping, as its invigorating effect may keep you awake. Follow with a warm then cold shower to improve circulation and elimination, moving the shower head from the feet upwards. Finish the shower by running cold or tepid water over the base of your skull and down your spine for 30 seconds; this will allow your glandular system, nervous system and other organs to work much more efficiently and can even stop you from getting colds. Skin brushing is excellent for exfoliation, since it removes dead surface skin layers along with other toxins, metabolic wastes and bacteria shed by cells. It keeps our pores unclogged and improves the skin's elimination ability.

EXERCISE TO KEEP LYMPH MOVING

As explained in Step Four, we have more lymph in our body than we have blood; however, the lymph does not have a pump and relies on us taking deep diaphragmatic breaths and moving a lot to allow it to move around the body. Muscle movement and gravity are meant to keep lymph flowing, pump lymph back through its channels and eliminate waste. Running and other forms of aerobic exercise encourage correct lymph activity and flush wastes from tissue fluids.

Using a rebounder (a mini trampoline) for just a few minutes daily is excellent for promoting correct lymph movement. We eliminate through our skin, lungs, kidneys and colon. Up to a third of waste elimination is through the skin, however, and our sweat glands should expel a minimum of 450g (1lb) of waste material daily. When they don't, because our bodies are not working at peak efficiency, this toxic waste can remain in our system causing all kinds of damage.

PERFECT SKIN CARE

Our skin is the largest organ in the body. It has two-way elimination and uses perspiration to flush elements out of our bodies and is able to absorb other elements through itself by means of sunshine, aromatherapy oils, herbal rubs and balms, and so on. After the brain, the skin is the most complex organ. It is comprised of, among other things, nerve endings, blood vessels, sweat glands, muscles, sensory cells and receptors that respond to heat, cold and touch – as well as responding wonderfully to skin brushing. Skin brushing regularly for only a few minutes daily can be as effective as 30 minutes of exercise, because it improves physical tone and muscle tone. However, you need to do it in addition to exercise, not in place of it. It has a very important place in making us feel and look years younger while improving our sense of well-being. It is so very easy to do and will soon become an automatic part of your morning routine, because the benefits easily outweigh the small investment of time required to skin brush properly. Here's how to start:

- You must use a natural vegetable-bristle brush found in most health-food shops and chemists.
- Skin brushing is best done in the morning prior to showering.
- Your body and the brush must be dry.

Exercise 17: How to skin brush

1 Beginning with the soles of your feet, brush in between the toes, then brush vigorously up your legs, front and back, using firm, sweeping strokes.

2 From the thighs, brush towards the groin, which is the major lymph gland and store.

3 Over the stomach, brush in a circular clockwise movement following the natural line of the colon. Repeat about ten times.

4 Brush the palms of your hands and then the backs, then move up the arms and shoulders.

5 Brush upwards towards the heart, then downwards once you are above the heart.

6 Brush downwards over the neck, throat and chest, then brush your upper and lower back and bottom.

7 Always avoid the nipples, groin and very irritated or infected skin, as well as severe varicose veins and the face, although you can get special softer brushes for facial brushing from most chemists or beauty shops. ▶

---

8   You can brush the scalp to stimulate hair growth and to improve the hair's texture and condition.

9   Brush more gently initially and more firmly over time. In the beginning, do it daily for three months, then several times each week.

10   Spend about five minutes on skin brushing and follow with a hot shower, ending it with a few moments of cold water – or lukewarm, if you can't bear the cold spray.

11   Look after your body brush by washing it once a week using natural soap, rinse it thoroughly, dry it naturally and don't share it with anyone.

Taking a bath with Epsom salts, bicarbonate of soda and root ginger helps the body to eliminate toxins by activating toxin movement in the tissues and increasing perspiration. Add two cups of Epsom salts, one cup of bicarbonate of soda and a cube of root ginger to the bath.

Saunas help you to sweat and this, in turn, flushes toxins and heavy metals out of your body while increasing cardiovascular activity.

Sleep and ageing

Proper sleep is essential if you want to age well. Not only is the correct amount of sleep vital but when and how you sleep are also important. Cells repair and regenerate at night. It has been said that humans sleep so that the process of cell regeneration can be carried out. Animals that have a shorter lifespan and don't have any cell turnover don't sleep at all; for example, butterflies, insects and deer.

Cell regeneration seems to occur at around 2.00 a.m., so it is important to be asleep by that time on most nights. Staying up late on a regular basis is very ageing; it has been said that one hour of sleep before midnight is equivalent to two hours of sleep after.

ABIDE BY YOUR BODY CLOCK

We are all cyclical by nature, and our body has its own clock – a good example of this is the menstrual cycle. Our body clock is designed to do certain things at certain times so, for example, exercise is better taken in the morning, digestion is better in the afternoon and sleep is better at night. It is fine to have some late nights and to stay up late having fun, but make sure you compensate for that by having some early nights and sleeping well at other times. It is hard for the body to catch up on lost sleep, and the body functions much better with consistent patterns of sleep rather than with sleep patterns that are erratic and constantly changing. Regular sleep is needed so that the brain can stay alert and function efficiently.

Females who have to work through the night, such as casino staff, nurses, airline staff, the police force and members of the emergency services, can be more prone to hormonal problems, erratic periods and conception problems, and this has been tied to the fact that the body's natural rhythms become disturbed. Night workers have a higher record of colds and depression, and a much weaker immune system, because the body never truly adapts to the reversing of the sleeping and waking cycle. We are meant to sleep when it's dark and rise when it's light.

If you want to have great skin and consistent energy, and to look and feel younger, you must have enough sleep and at the right time of night too – this becomes even more important as we get older.

THE SLEEP WRINKLES

Even the way you sleep can have an effect on your skin. A wrinkle is a crease in the skin that occurs when the collagen beneath the skin's layer is imprinted by a continual muscle action such as frowning, smiling, squinting, grimacing, and so on. People with facial paralysis often have unlined skin, because they don't have these muscle actions. Many people sleep in a way that causes their face, their skin, to 'pleat' while they sleep. By nature we appear to sleep more on our right side than our left and some people notice they have slightly more, or more deeply pronounced lines and wrinkles on their right side. If you sleep on your stomach or with your face pressed into a pillow, this will leave a wrinkle memory in your skin – in other words a premature wrinkle that could have been avoided.

Sleeping with a lot of pillows makes this much worse; sleep with only one pillow and choose a pillow that is quite flat. A foam memory pillow is best if you have been used to two or three plump, squashy pillows, you will miss them at first but then not even notice the difference. It is best to sleep on your back or side with your pillow under your neck and head if you wish to avoid lines and wrinkles. Using a pure silk pillowcase helps to avoid the facial 'pleating' that occurs while sleeping.

If you don't find it easy to get to sleep quickly, put some lavender oil on your pillow, which is very relaxing. Alternatively, playing one of the downloads from this programme, which are intended to be played prior to sleeping at night, will make you very relaxed and send you to sleep.

SLEEP GUIDELINES

To help you enjoy better sleep:

- Sleep in a room that is well ventilated.

- Don't sleep with the heating on, unless it is exceptionally cold.
- Don't sleep with your head by a radiator or close to electrical appliances, because of the effects of electro-magnetic rays passing into your body during the night (see page 246).
- Don't overstimulate your mind just before bed by watching scary films or reading frightening novels, if you don't sleep well.
- Don't overstimulate your mind by working on a computer before bed.
- Don't eat a lot of food before going to bed, because digesting late at night prevents the body from fully resting.

Activity – a perfect way to become younger

Here is your final exercise for looking and feeling younger.

Exercise 18: Take action around the home

1   Go through the list of wonder-foods on pages 216–26 and choose the ones you intend to buy. Make sure you regularly include wonder-foods in your shopping and menus, and choose these foods whenever you eat out.

2   Go through your fridge and cupboards and eliminate trans fats and unhealthy artificial sweeteners from your home.

▶

---

3 List the vitamins (see page 232) that you need to take and ensure you order or purchase a regular supply.

4 Decide how you can exercise, and make it a lifelong part of your lifestyle. Find a class to go to regularly, exercise with a friend or use an exercise DVD. Make exercising a compulsive habit. Even walking further instead of driving, and taking the stairs rather than the lift, will make a difference over time.

5 Move any electrical appliances in your bedroom away from the area around your bed. Take some appliances out of the room, or at least put them on the floor away from your pillows as you sleep.

6 Put plants behind your computer and move the seating in your home further away from the television, sound system and radiators. Re-install your normal handset telephones and use them more often than your cordless or mobile phones.

7 Buy digestive enzymes (page 238) and a body brush (page 262), and take them, or use them, regularly.

8 Take away surplus pillows or put them on the floor while you are sleeping (page 265).

You will find making these lifestyle changes easy and will also find yourself making more of them, because the results you get will be so visible and you will feel so much better that you will become more motivated to continue making them a part of your life.

The Common Denominators of 100-year-olds

Many tests have been done on centenarians to find out the secrets of those who live to be 100 years old or more. The tests are quite diverse and often have conflicting information. However, it is becoming easier to study people of 100 years of age because every year there are more of them to study. In 1951 there were 300 100-year-olds in Britain; by 2012 the figure was 12,320, with 610 thought to be aged 105 or over. The Office for National Statistics has also noted a rise in people living to 110, although in analysing the age at which death is most common, the ONS found most men are living until they are 85, and women to 89.

There is no doubt that we are living longer, and being 100 years old will become absolutely routine as people go beyond the age of 100 by many more years. Genes will be only partly to do with this, since even if both your parents live long lives that may add only about three years to your life. Having parents who live long lives, however, will increase your expectation of doing the same.

Full lives, natural diets

In numerous tests carried out on centenarians in Japan, America and Europe, the common denominators that they shared were a feeling of being loved, of feeling respected, valued and appreciated. They all had some degree of independence, they had usually worked hard throughout their lives and took an active interest in life in general and in their life in particular. On the whole they wanted to go on living and had a reason to do so. The studies on their diet were vastly different, but they had obviously eaten less processed and chemically treated food when they were younger. This is a relatively recent addition to food, and centenarians' diets consisted of much more natural food – predominantly vegetables, fruits, grains and protein – and significantly less sugar and snacks. Another common denominator was that almost all the centenarians had not overeaten. Some of them had smoked but they had been exposed to less pollution in general.

Many societies and groups of longer-living old people eat a diet that includes foods such as yoghurt, apricots, oily fish and honey. In his book *Seven Health Secrets From the Hive*, Charles Robson documents tribes where people are chronologically very old yet actually stay very young and healthy on diets rich in bee pollen, propolis and royal jelly (see page 222).

Physical activity and a strong mind

Activity was a trait all the centenarians shared. They had all been active, they had all worked hard – often at some form of manual labour – and in their younger years, of course, housework was hard manual work. Many of them still did some housework or cooking, and they had usually enjoyed a healthy sex life, which many of them continued into their eighties. When you keep your sex life going, your body assumes you must be doing this to procreate, whatever age you are, and this in turn boosts anti-ageing. When you orgasm, you make natural killer (NK) cells that fight illness and age-related illnesses, helping you to look and feel younger. Having regular orgasms helps you to live longer. A study conducted at Wilkes University in Pennsylvania discovered that one or two orgasms per week can increase the body's infection-fighting cells by up to a third. The American Longevity Project showed that women who have more orgasms live longer.

The centenarians mentioned above were mentally active too and stimulated their brains by being involved in activities and maintaining an interest in current affairs. They had hobbies and were interested in what was going on around them. They remained curious and had a good sense of humour, laughed a lot, still had fun and did not feel that they were a burden to others. They shared in common a vitality, energy and radiance about life, they were generally optimistic, were positive in their attitude and were happy and fulfilled.

What these tests of 'young old people' from around the world show is that personality, especially a strong and positive personality, is as strong a factor in staying young as making changes in your health. Reports from the Medical Research Council show that wilful, cantankerous old people can live longer. Similar studies with chronic illness show the same wilful cantankerous character has a high disposition to survive illness at any age. A desire not to conform or be passive is talked about in Dr Bernie Siegal's book *Love, Medicine and Miracles*, in which he says that if you want to survive a chronic illness have the word 'uncooperative' written on your medical notes.

Conclusion

Well done for finishing this book, but this is not an ending, it's a new beginning. From start to finish of this book I have described absorbing, powerful and workable solutions to becoming and staying younger. You cannot adhere to this programme without seeing and feeling the benefits. As long as you use this book in the way it was intended, you can age agelessly. You will already think differently now, and you have begun a process to achieve your goals so that you can remain younger.

You have learned how to change your thoughts, your beliefs, your language – and even your physiology – in the area of ageing. You have also learned how to make affirmations work for you and how to become a physical expression of your affirmations. You have been shown how to program your mind to age excellently, how to visualise being younger and how to reclaim and redefine a wonderful, positive and ageless image of yourself. You have taken physical tests to prove that you have power over your body and no outside source can influence and affect your body to the extent that you can. You have tested your biological age and you can refer to the tests for ageing successfully again and again, each time noticing how much better your score is, especially as you have learned to use the anti-ageing properties of vitamins, exercise and certain foods. Finally, you learned that moving electrical appliances, using skin brushing and enjoying proper sleep and digestion can allow you to live years longer while looking years younger. You have learned new thinking and this can become, for you, a lifelong habit, you can move on from one great achievement to another in the area of staying young. You have discovered that small changes can give you big results and that this is not some New Age hocus-pocus – it is a science that really works.

The exercises are the core of this book

It's essential that you have not only read this book from cover to cover but that you have also worked through all the exercises required. (If you have skipped any of them, please go back and do them right now – not for me, but for you.) I designed these exercises so that you can communicate with your cells, making changes that are physical and mental so that you change on the inside as well as on the outside. You may find yourself wanting to read this book or favourite parts of it again, and I recommend that you do so. It is a very good idea to return to the programme perhaps every six months, or every time you celebrate another birthday, and do some refresher exercises to remind yourself that you can choose how young you want to feel and be.

Your life will be changed forever

Congratulations for staying with the book. I applaud you for doing all the work. The rewards you will get from the investment you made by fully participating in this programme are endless. It's up to you to implement these changes and to continue with this new way of thinking, this new belief system and attitude and these new habits and lifestyle changes.

The part I love the most about my programme is that you don't have to do all of it all the time for it to work. As long as you do most of it most of the time, it will work. It's down to you to go on making the changes work for you in all aspects of your life and, of course, to believe and know you can do it.

As long as you do this you cannot, and will not, return to your old ways of thinking and feeling.

A positive mental attitude

It is also vital to be calm and positive and to always have an optimistic view of ageing, since to age well we need to be free from panic, we need to be calm, to have unshakeable confidence and conviction in our body's ability to regenerate itself, to bring about its own healing and repair. To know and believe that we can stay younger at any age. I know that you can do it.

You will get ill and tired much less if you feel good about yourself and take full responsibility for how you feel – not just now but all the time. You will age remarkably better if you feel happy, so it really is important to laugh every day, to have a sense of humour, to be childlike and not always to take things and life too seriously. People have cured themselves of illness by something called laughter therapy, which involves laughing daily. Norman Cousins, in his book *Anatomy of an Illness as Perceived by the Patient*, describes the techniques he used to cure himself of chronic illness. These included installing a video and television in his room and renting as many funny films and series as he could and laughing for hours every day, which caused his body to make the healing chemicals he needed to fight the disease.

So what next?

You have been through a process – a powerful process – and you have worked hard to make powerful, lasting changes. They won't undo themselves, and if you are at all worried that they will, remember you have an additional special tool – your downloaded recordings.

Repetition is called the mother of all skills. Remember that I told you that repeating actions creates a neural pathway to the brain that is reinforced with every repetition. When you listen to the downloads and see yourself as younger, you are sending messages to your subconscious mind that will further help you to become this way. You will be continuously reinforcing all the good changes you are making until they stick and you are rewired to slow down ageing. The recordings are going to help you so much. They will have a powerful, permanent and all-pervasive impact on you, so play them every day without a break for 21 days (remember those neural pathways change after 21 days) and then continue to play them regularly until the words become deeply embedded and encoded into your subconscious mind.

I hope you have enjoyed this journey to be younger. The destination is fantastic – it's you looking and feeling great whatever your years, living a longer, healthier and younger life. Make sure you enjoy the process, and please let me know how you have changed and what has happened to you since you became a participant in the philosophy of *You Can be Younger*. I love hearing from people who have benefited from this process, so please email me via my website at www.marisapeer.com, or contact me for advice. Perhaps you will become a part of my next book.

I have so enjoyed writing this book and showing you the things that have made a huge difference in my life and that of my clients. Thank you so much for taking this journey with me. Perhaps I will meet you one day at one of my seminars, I hope so.

Here's looking at (the new younger) you.

With love from,

Marisa Peer.

Notes

1 W. Evans and I. Rosenberg, *Biomarkers*, Simon & Schuster, 1991
2 P. Anversa et al., 'Bone marrow cells regenerate infarcted myocardium', *Nature*, 2001;410: 701–5
3 J. Frisen et al., 'Identification of a neural stem cell in the adult mammalian central nervous system', *Cell*, 1999;96(1):25–34
4 H. Beecher, *Research and the Individual: Human Studies*, Little, Brown (Boston), 1970
5 In a recent study of a new kind of chemotherapy, 30 per cent of the individuals in the control group, the group given placebos, lost their hair, C. Evans, *Cancer Uncensored*, 2012
6 D. Ornish et al., 'Effect of comprehensive lifestyle changes on telomerase activity and telomere length in men with biopsy-proven low-risk prostate cancer: 5-year follow-up of a descriptive pilot study', *The Lancet Oncology*, 2013;14(11):1112–20
7 L. Olivia et al., 'High phobic anxiety is related to lower leukocyte telomere length in women', *PLoS One*, 2012;7(7):e40515. Epub Jul 11, 2012
8 T. L. Jacobs et al., 'Intensive meditation training, immune cell telomerase activity, and psychological mediators', *Psychoneuroendocrinology*, 2011;35(5):664–81
9 D. Chopra, Ageless Body, Timeless Mind, Rider, 2008
10 Research at the Dutch National Institute of Public Health found that of 800 elderly Dutch men, those consuming a steady supply of quercetin had a 60 per cent reduced risk of heart attack. M. Hertog and P. Hollman, 'Potential health effects of the dietary flavonol quercetin', *European Journal of Clinical Nutrition*, 1996;50(2):63–71
11 C. Secor and D. Lisk, 'Variation in the selenium content of individual Brazil nuts', *Journal of Food Safety*, 1989;9(4):279–81

12 Research at the Strang-Cornell Cancer Research Laboratory in New York City found 70 per cent of women eating cabbage began burning off dangerous oestrogen within five days. M. Osborne et al., 'Upregulation of estradiol C16α-hydroxylation in human breast tissue: a potential biomarker of breast cancer risk', *Journal of the National Cancer Institute*, 1993;85(23):1917–20

13 J. Morris et al., 'Effects of garlic extract on platelet aggregation: a randomized placebo-controlled double-blind study', *Clinical and Experimental Pharmacology and Physiology*, 1995;22(6–7):414–17

14 K. Srivastava, 'Effect of onion and ginger consumption on platelet thromboxane production in humans', *Prostaglandins, Leukotrienes and Essential Fatty Acids*, 1989;

    35(3):183–5; Dr Tariq Mustafa associate professor at The Institute of Biology, Odense found ginger to inhibit two of the enzymes responsible for inflammation and arthritis, 'Biological basis for the use of botanicals in osteoarthritis and rheutamoid arthritis: a review', *Evidence-Based Complementary and Alternative Medicine*, 2005; 2(3):301–8

15 Research at the University of Wisconsin demonstrated that three glasses of purple/red grape juice have an anti-clogging effect on arteries. 'Purple grape juice improves endothelial function and reduces the susceptibility of LDL cholesterol to oxidation in patients with coronary artery disease', *Circulation*, 1999;100(10):1050–55

16 Studies in Germany and Italy have shown the benefits of tomatoes and dietary fibre.

    'Dietary fibre in food and protection against colorectal cancer in the European Prospective Investigation into Cancer and Nutrition (EPIC): an observational study', *The Lancet*, 2003; 361(9368):1496–1501

17 'Hopes Rising For Selenium', Dr Donald Lisk, Professor of Toxicology at Cornell University, the *New York Times*, February 19, 1997; *see also* S. Lippman, 'Effect of selenium and vitamin E on risk of prostate cancer and other cancers: The Selenium and Vitamin E Cancer Prevention Trial (SELECT)', *Journal of the American Medical Association*, 2009;301(1):39–51

18 J. Kleijnen and P. Knipschild, 'Ginkgo biloba for cerebral insufficiency', *British Journal of Clinical Pharmacology*, 1992; 34(4):352–8